Foot and Ankle Injuries and Treatment

Editors

ANISH R. KADAKIA
JOSEPH S. PARK

CLINICS IN
SPORTS MEDICINE

www.sportsmed.theclinics.com

Consulting Editor
MARK D. MILLER

October 2020 • Volume 39 • Number 4

ELSEVIER

1600 John F. Kennedy Boulevard • Suite 1800 • Philadelphia, Pennsylvania, 19103-2899

http://www.theclinics.com

CLINICS IN SPORTS MEDICINE Volume 39, Number 4
October 2020 ISSN 0278-5919, ISBN-13: 978-0-323-75500-9

Editor: Lauren Boyle
Developmental Editor: Donald Mumford

Clinics in Sports Medicine (ISSN 0278-5919) is published quarterly by Elsevier Inc., 360 Park Avenue South, New York, NY 10010-1710. Months of issue are January, April, July, and October. Business and Editorial Offices: 1600 John F. Kennedy Blvd., Ste. 1800, Philadelphia, PA 19103-2899. Customer Service Office: 3251 Riverport Lane, Maryland Heights, MO 63043. Periodicals postage paid at New York, NY and additional mailing offices. Subscription prices are $364.00 per year (US individuals), $733.00 per year (US institutions), $100.00 per year (US students), $405.00 per year (Canadian individuals), $904.00 per year (Canadian institutions), $100.00 (Canadian students), $475.00 per year (foreign individuals), $904.00 per year (foreign institutions), and $235.00 per year (foreign students). Foreign air speed delivery is included in all *Clinics* subscription prices. All prices are subject to change without notice. **POSTMASTER:** Send address changes to *Clinics in Sports Medicine*, Elsevier Health Sciences Division, Subscription Customer Service, 3251 Riverport Lane, Maryland Heights, MO 63043. Customer Service (orders, claims, online, change of address): Elsevier Health Sciences Division, Subscription Customer Service, 3251 Riverport Lane, Maryland Heights, MO 63043. **Tel: 1-800-654-2452 (U.S. and Canada); 314-447-8871 (outside U.S. and Canada). Fax: 314-447-8029. E-mail: journalscustomerservice-usa@elsevier.com (for print support); journalsonlinesupport-usa@ elsevier.com (for online support).**

Reprints. For copies of 100 or more of articles in this publication, please contact the Commercial Reprints Department, Elsevier Inc., 360 Park Avenue South, New York, NY 10010-1710. Tel.: 212-633-3874; Fax: 212-633-3820; E-mail: reprints@elsevier.com.

Clinics in Sports Medicine is covered in *MEDLINE/PubMed (Index Medicus) Current Contents/Clinical Medicine, Excerpta Medica,* and *ISI/Biomed.*

Contributors

CONSULTING EDITOR

MARK D. MILLER, MD
S. Ward Casscells Professor, Head, Department of Orthopaedic Surgery, Division of Sports Medicine, University of Virginia, Charlottesville, Virginia, USA; Team Physician, Miller Review Course, Harrisonburg, Virginia, USA

EDITORS

ANISH R. KADAKIA, MD
Professor of Orthopedic Surgery–Foot and Ankle, Program Director, Foot and Ankle Orthopedic Fellowship, Center for Comprehensive Orthopaedic and Spine Care, Northwestern University Feinberg School of Medicine, Department of Orthopedic Surgery, Northwestern Memorial Hospital, Chicago, Illinois, USA

JOSEPH S. PARK, MD
Associate Professor, Department of Orthopedic Surgery, Foot and Ankle Division Head, University of Virginia Health System, Charlottesville, Virginia, USA

AUTHORS

AMIETHAB A. AIYER, MD
Chief, Foot and Ankle Service, Department of Orthopaedics, University of Miami Miller School of Medicine, Miami, Florida, USA

MOHAMMED T. ALSHOULI, MD
Deputy Chairman of the Orthopedic Department, Prince Mohammed Bin AbdulAziz Hospital, Visiting Professor and Clinical Instructor, Imam Bin Saud University, College of Medicine, Clinical Professor and Clinical Instructor, Dar Aloloom University, College of Medicine, Riyadh, Saudi Arabia

MAURICIO P. BARBOSA, MD
Orthobone Clinic, Asccociaiacao Beneficente Siria HCor, Sao Paul, Brazil

STEVE B. BEHRENS, MD
Assistant Attending Orthopedic Surgeon, Hospital for Special Surgery, Weill Cornell Medical College, New York, New York, USA

DANIEL BRIGGS, MD
Department of Orthopedic Surgery, Center for Comprehensive Orthopaedic and Spine Care, Northwestern Memorial Hospital, Chicago, Illinois, USA

JOHN T. CAMPBELL, MD
Director of Research, Institute for Foot and Ankle Reconstruction, Mercy Medical Center, Clinical Associate Professor, Department of Orthopaedics, University of Maryland School of Medicine, Baltimore, Maryland, USA

MICHAEL J. CASALE, MD
Attending Orthopedic Surgeon, Raleigh Orthopedic Clinic, Foot and Ankle Surgery, Raleigh, North Carolina, USA

MATTHEW S. CONTI, MD
Orthopaedic Surgery Resident, Hospital for Special Surgery, Weill Cornell Medical College, New York, New York, USA

MINTON TRUITT COOPER, MD
Associate Professor, Department of Orthopaedic Surgery, University of Virginia, Charlottesvlle, Virginia, USA

J. KENT ELLINGTON, MD, MS
OrthoCarolina Foot & Ankle Institute, Charlotte, North Carolina, USA

ERIC FERKEL, MD
Attending Orthopedic Surgeon, Southern California Orthopedic Institute, Van Nuys, California, USA

JAVIER GUZMAN, MD
Department of Orthopaedic Surgery, Icahn School of Medicine at Mount Sinai, New York, New York, USA

CLIFFORD L. JENG, MD
Medical Director, Institute for Foot and Ankle Reconstruction, Mercy Medical Center, Baltimore, Maryland, USA

CARROLL P. JONES, MD
OrthoCarolina Foot & Ankle Institute, Fellowship Director, Associate Professor, Atrium MSK Institute, Charlotte, North Carolina, USA

ANISH R. KADAKIA, MD
Professor of Orthopedic Surgery–Foot and Ankle, Program Director, Foot and Ankle Orthopedic Fellowship, Center for Comprehensive Orthopaedic and Spine Care, Northwestern University Feinberg School of Medicine, Department of Orthopedic Surgery, Northwestern Memorial Hospital, Chicago, Illinois, USA

JOSHUA T. KAISER, BS
Medical Student - MS3, University of Miami Miller School of Medicine, Miami, Florida, USA

JOHN Y. KWON, MD
Chief, Orthopaedic Foot and Ankle Service, Department of Orthopaedic Surgery, Associate Professor, Harvard Medical School, Beth Israel Deaconess Medical Center, Boston, Massachusetts, USA

CORY KWONG, MD
Sports Medicine Surgery and Arthroscopy Fellow, Southern California Orthopedic Institute, Van Nuys, California, USA

JULIAN G. LUGO-PICO, MD
Orthopaedic Surgery, PGY5, University of Miami, Jackson Memorial Hospital, Miami, Florida, USA

MUHAMMAD Y. MUTAWAKKIL, MD
Department of Orthopedic Surgery, Northwestern Memorial Hospital, Center for Comprehensive Orthopaedic and Spine Care, Chicago, Illinois, USA

SHAWN NGUYEN, DO
Sports Medicine Surgery and Arthroscopy Fellow, Southern California Orthopedic Institute, Van Nuys, California, USA

JEFFREY OKEWUNMI, BS
Department of Orthopaedic Surgery, Icahn School of Medicine at Mount Sinai, New York, New York, USA

JOSEPH S. PARK, MD
Associate Professor, Department of Orthopedic Surgery, Foot and Ankle Division Head, University of Virginia Health System, Charlottesville, Virginia, USA

MILAP S. PATEL, DO
Department of Orthopedic Surgery, Northwestern Memorial Hospital, Center for Comprehensive Orthopaedic and Spine Care, Chicago, Illinois, USA

RAFAEL A. SANCHEZ, MD
Orthopaedic Surgery, PGY4, University of Miami, Jackson Memorial Hospital, Miami, Florida, USA

B. DALE SHARPE, DO
Resident, Residency Program, OhioHealth Orthopedic Surgery, Columbus, Ohio, USA

BRIAN D. STEGINSKY, DO
Attending Orthopedic Surgeon, OhioHealth Orthopedic Surgeons, Columbus, Ohio, USA

DEREK S. STENQUIST, MD
Harvard Combined Orthopaedic Residency Program, Boston, Massachusetts, USA

MALLORY SUHLING, BS
Foot and Ankle Research Coordinator, Illinois Bone and Joint Institute, LLC, Libertyville, Illinois, USA

ANAND VORA, MD
Attending Orthopedic Surgeon, Illinois Bone and Joint Institute, LLC, Libertyville, Illinois, USA

ETTORE VULCANO, MD
Department of Orthopaedic Surgery, Icahn School of Medicine at Mount Sinai, New York, New York, USA

MICHAEL Y. YE, BSE
Research Assistant, Department of Orthopaedic Surgery, Beth Israel Deaconess Medical Center, Boston, Massachusetts, USA

MUHAMMAD Y. MUTAWAKKIL, MO
Department of Orthopaedic Surgery, Northwestern Memorial Hospital
Comprehensive Orthopaedic and Spine Care, Chicago, Illinois, USA

Contents

> Despite the fact that ankle fractures are common injuries, not all patients obtain satisfactory results. Historically, the deltoid ligament injury and intra-articular pathology have not often been treated at the time of fracture stabilization. Recent literature has suggested that repair of the deltoid ligament may lead to better stability of the ankle mortise. Additionally, the use of arthroscopy in conjunction with fracture fixation may allow for better identification and treatment of intra-articular lesions and improve detection and reduction of subtle instability.

> Acute and chronic syndesmotic injuries significantly impact athletic function and activities of daily living. Patient history, examination, and judicious use of imaging modalities aid diagnosis. Surgical management should be used when frank diastasis, instability, and/or chronic pain and disability ensue. Screw and suture-button fixation remain the mainstay of treatment of acute injuries, but novel syndesmotic reconstruction techniques hold promise for treatment of acute and chronic injuries, especially for athletes. This article focuses on anatomy, mechanisms of injury, diagnosis, and surgical reduction and stabilization of acute and chronic syndesmotic instability. Fixation methods with a focus on considerations for athletes are discussed.

> Lisfranc injuries can be devastating to the athlete and nonathlete. In the athletic population, minor loss of midfoot stability compromises the high level of function demanded of the lower extremity. The most critical aspect of treatment is identifying the injury and severity of the ligamentous/articular damage. Not all athletes are able to return to their previous level of function. With appropriate treatment, a Lisfranc injury does not mandate the cessation of an athletic career. We focus on the diagnosis and an algorithmic approach to treatment in the athlete discussion the controversy of open reduction and internal fixation versus arthrodesis.

recommended to address intra-articular disorder before stabilization. An anatomic approach provides full range of motion, stability, and return to sport and activity. Allograft or suture tape augmentation can be useful for patients with generalized ligamentous laxity, patients with high body mass index, and elite athletes. Allograft reconstruction may be especially useful in revision procedures. Arthroscopic approach to lateral ankle ligament stabilization may provide good outcomes, with long-term data still limited.

Peroneal tendinosis and subluxation are lifestyle-limiting conditions that can worsen if not properly diagnosed and treated. Adequate knowledge of ankle anatomy and detailed history and comprehensive physical examination is essential for diagnosis. Peroneal tendinopathy is likely to result from overuse, whereas subluxation often precipitates from forceful contraction of peroneals during sudden dorsiflexion while landing or abruptly stopping. In athletes, conservative measures remain first-line treatment of tendinopathy, but surgery is often immediately indicated in cases of recurrent symptomatic subluxation or dislocation. Surgical technique varies on the type, mechanism, and severity of injury, but most procedures have a high success rate.

Painful accessory navicular and spring ligament injuries in athletes are different entities from more common posterior tibialis tendon problems seen in older individuals. These injuries typically affect running and jumping athletes, causing medial arch pain and in severe cases a pes planus deformity. Diagnosis requires a detailed physical examination, standing radiographs, and MRI. Initial treatment focuses on rest, immobilization, and restriction from sports. Orthotic insoles may alleviate minor pain, but many patients need surgery to expedite recovery and return to sports. The authors review their approach to these injuries and provide surgical tips along with expected rehabilitation to provide optimal outcomes.

Recreational athletes are susceptible to experiencing pain in the Achilles tendon, affecting their ability to complete daily activities. Achilles tendinosis is a degenerative process of the tendon without histologic or clinical signs of intratendinous inflammation, which can be categorized by location into insertional and noninsertional tendinosis. This condition is one that can be treated conservatively with great success or surgically for refractory cases. Currently, there is a lack of consensus regarding the best treatment options. This review aims to explore both conservative and operative treatment options for Achilles tendinopathy and Achilles tendon rupture.

Surgical management of osteochondral lesions of the talus without an osteotomy depends on the size, location, and chronicity of the lesion. Bone
marrow stimulation techniques, such as microfracture, can be performed
arthroscopically and have consistently good outcomes in lesions less than
1 cm in diameter. For lesions not amenable to bone marrow stimulation,
one-stage techniques, such as allograft cartilage extracellular matrix and
allograft juvenile hyaline cartilage, may be used. Arthroscopy may be
used in many cases to address these lesions; however, an arthrotomy
may be required to use osteochondral autograft and allograft transplantation techniques.

Posterior ankle pain is a common complaint, and the potential causative
pathologic processes are diverse. The constellation of these numerous etiologies has been collectively referred to as posterior ankle impingement
syndrome. The pain associated with posterior ankle impingement is
caused by bony or soft tissue impingement of the posterior ankle while
in terminal plantar flexion. This condition is most frequently encountered
in athletes who participate in sports that involve forceful, or repetitive,
ankle plantar flexion. This article discusses the associated pathology,
diagnosis, conservative treatment, and surgical techniques associated
with flexor hallucis longus and posterior ankle impingement syndrome.

CLINICS IN SPORTS MEDICINE

SERIES OF RELATED INTERESTED

Orthopedic Clinics
Foot and Ankle Clinics
Hand Clinics
Physical Medicine and Rehabilitation Clinics

THE CLINICS ARE AVAILABLE ONLINE!
Access your subscription at:
www.theclinics.com

Foreword

Best Foot Foreword

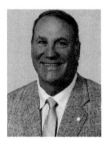

Mark D. Miller, MD
Consulting Editor

It is a pleasure to introduce this issue of *Clinics in Sports Medicine* on Foot and Ankle Injuries and Treatment. I learned early in my sports medicine career that it is important to have a skilled foot and ankle surgeon on your team. Injuries to this area are common, and a special understanding of not only foot and ankle injuries but specifically sports foot and ankle injuries is critical for the successful management of these athletes. I am honored to have worked with many excellent foot and ankle surgeons, and the 2 coeditors of this issue of *Clinics in Sports Medicine* are no exception. I have been partners with Dr Park since his arrival at UVA 10 years ago. With his partners, he has taken care of athletes from the 2 major universities that we have the pleasure to serve, and he has been involved in numerous cases of knee dislocation with associated nerve injuries. I have also been lucky to have known and worked with Dr Kadakia for almost as long through numerous academic pursuits.

This issue covers the gambit of sports foot and ankle injuries. Excellent articles on fractures, ligament injuries, tendon injuries, and articular cartilage injuries are all included. I appreciate the "shout out" from both of the editors, but having been a guest editor myself, I assure you that they have "footed" the lion's share of the work. Thank

Clin Sports Med 39 (2020) xiii–xiv
https://doi.org/10.1016/j.csm.2020.07.009
0278-5919/20/© 2020 Published by Elsevier Inc.

sportsmed.theclinics.com

you to the guest editors for putting together a great treatise on treating foot and ankle injuries in athletes.

Mark D. Miller, MD
Division of Sports Medicine
Department of Orthopaedic Surgery
University of Virginia
James Madison University
400 Ray C. Hunt Drive, Suite 330
Charlottesville, VA 22908-0159, USA

E-mail address:
MDM3P@hscmail.mcc.virginia.edu

Preface

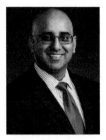 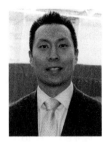

Anish R. Kadakia, MD   Joseph S. Park, MD
Editors

When we were asked to be guest editors for this Foot and Ankle issue of *Clinics in Sports Medicine*, we appreciated the magnitude of this amazing opportunity to share the expertise of our Orthopedic Foot and Ankle community with our Sports Medicine colleagues around the country. Just as our Sports Medicine colleagues have revolutionized ACL reconstruction, cartilage regeneration, arthroscopy, and rotator cuff repair, our Foot and Ankle members have led the charge for advancing syndesmotic fixation, surgical treatment of ankle instability and turf toe injuries, tendon transfers for foot drop, and innovative approaches to fracture fixation and tendon repair. As we are both fortunate to work closely with athletes of all levels, we have been amazed and humbled to watch many of our players return to the playing field after sustaining career-threatening foot and ankle injuries.

Our subspecialty has continued to play an increasingly critical role in the evaluation and treatment of collegiate and professional athletes, and we are honored to be a small part of the team that cares for these patients. Collaboration between Sports Medicine and Foot and Ankle Orthopedic Surgeons is the key to improving the care we can deliver to our athletic patient population.

We have carefully enlisted some of the true leaders in our field to contribute to this Special Foot and Ankle issue of *Clinics in Sports Medicine*, and we would like to thank the authors for their dedication and time taken away from family. We hope that like us, you will learn from these in-depth reviews of these carefully curated foot and ankle topics specifically focused on the athlete that challenge and frustrate us every day.

ACKNOWLEDGMENTS

Anish R. Kadakia, MD: My primary gratitude is to my wife Sakina and my four children, who have had to make the largest sacrifice in order to allow me to pursue my academic interests. A most heartfelt thank you to my co-editor Joseph Park, who helped make this issue come to fruition. My gratitude to all the authors who contributed to this issue for all their time away from family to write these well-researched and focused articles for the athlete. Thank you, Mark Miller, for the opportunity once again to be a part of a wonderful academic endeavor.

Joseph S. Park, MD: I would like to thank all of my teachers and mentors who have helped and guided me throughout my training and career. I am forever indebted to the Orthopedic Surgery faculty of NYU Hospital for Joint Diseases and to the remarkable Foot and Ankle Divisions at Union Memorial Hospital and Mercy Hospital in Baltimore. I am grateful to the many talented authors who made this issue possible, as well as my coeditor, Anish Kadakia, for taking on this challenge with me.

Thank you to my Chairman at the University of Virginia, Dr Bobby Chhabra, for your unwavering support of our Foot and Ankle Division and Fellowship, and to my Sports Medicine partners who have embraced the role our specialty takes in the care of our student athletes. I feel very fortunate to have talented physician and PA partners in the Foot and Ankle Division at UVA. A special thanks goes to the Consulting Editor of *Clinics in Sports Medicine*, Dr Mark Miller, a true giant in the world of Orthopedic Education.

I am eternally grateful to my parents and sisters, for their guidance and love. Finally, I want to thank my amazing wife, Ann Marie, who has supported me throughout this journey and has tolerated the long hours and last minute deadlines that always seem to encroach on our family life. Isabelle, Stephen, and Caroline are a testament to your dedication and patience as a mother, and I feel truly blessed every day.

Anish R. Kadakia, MD
Northwestern University
Feinberg School of Medicine
Department of Orthopedic Surgery
Northwestern Memorial Hospital
676 North St. Clair–Suite 1350
Chicago, IL 60611, USA

Joseph S. Park, MD
Department of Orthopedic Surgery
Foot and Ankle Division Head
University of Virginia Health System
400 Ray C. Hunt Drive
Suite 330
Charlottesville, VA 22908, USA

E-mail addresses:
kadak259@gmail.com (A.R. Kadakia)
jsp3x@virginia.edu (J.S. Park)

The Role of Deltoid Repair and Arthroscopy in Ankle Fractures

Minton Truitt Cooper, MD

KEYWORDS

- Ankle fracture • Ankle arthroscopy • Deltoid ligament • Syndesmosis
- Osteochondral lesion

KEY POINTS

- Despite the fact that deltoid ligament injuries are common in unstable ankle fractures, historically, this pathology has been neglected in treating these injuries.
- More recently, studies have described primary deltoid repair with excellent outcomes and improved stability of the ankle. Most of these have focused on repairing the anterior portion of the deltoid.
- Intra-articular pathology, such as chondral lesions, is extremely common in conjunction with unstable ankle fractures. Arthroscopy at the time of fracture fixation offers the ability to identify and treat these pathologies.
- Arthroscopy at the time of fracture fixation also offers the potential benefit of improved detection and treatment of subtle residual instability.

INTRODUCTION

Ankle fractures are among the most common injuries treated by orthopedic surgeons.[1,2] Recent advances in techniques and technology have changed the way many orthopedic conditions are treated, and ankle fractures are no exception. Historically, the treatment for an unstable ankle fracture with a deltoid injury has consisted primarily of repairing the fractured fibula and allowing the deltoid ligament injury to heal on its own. Although most patients treated in this manner obtain good results, there are still a subset of patients with poor outcomes, some of which may be caused by unrecognized additional injury.[3,4] This has led to an increase in interest of adjunct procedures when managing unstable ankle fractures, including arthroscopic procedures and repair of the deltoid ligament.

Department of Orthopaedic Surgery, University of Virginia, Box 800159, Charlottesvlle, VA 22908, USA
E-mail address: Mtc2d@virginia.edu

Clin Sports Med 39 (2020) 733–743
https://doi.org/10.1016/j.csm.2020.06.003
0278-5919/20/© 2020 Elsevier Inc. All rights reserved.
sportsmed.theclinics.com

ANATOMY OF THE DELTOID LIGAMENT

The ankle joint is often described as a mortise, with the talus maintained beneath the tibial plafond by the medial, lateral, and posterior malleoli, combined with the medial and lateral ankle ligaments. The syndesmotic structures including the anterior inferior tibiofibular ligament (AITFL), the posterior inferior tibiofibular ligament (PITFL), and the interosseous membrane/ligament stabilize the tibia and fibula distally, helping to preserve the congruence of this mortise.

The deltoid is an important medial stabilizer of the ankle joint.[5,6] Although many anatomic descriptions of the deltoid ligament complex have been suggested, it is agreed that it is composed of a superficial and deep portion.[7–9] The superficial deltoid arises from the anterior colliculus of the medial malleolus and attaches to the talus, navicular, sustentaculum of the calcaneus, and spring ligament (superficial posterior tibiotalar ligament, tibionavicular ligament, tibiocalcaneal ligament, and tibiospring ligament). The deep deltoid (deep anterior and posterior tibiotalar ligaments) arise from the interior margin of the posterior colliculus and insert on the medial talus.[8,10] (**Fig. 1**)

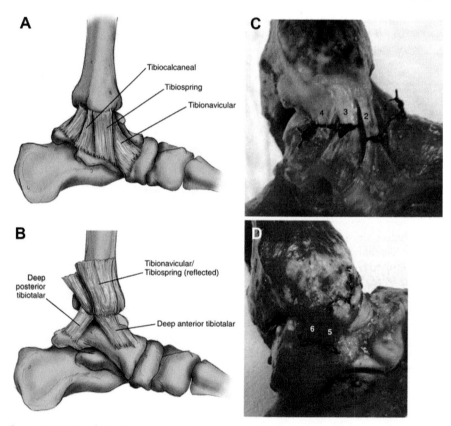

Fig. 1. Anatomy of the deltoid ligament complex. (*A*) The superficial deltoid. (*B*) Deep deltoid. (*C*) Cadaveric specimen showing the components of the superficial deltoid as discreet bands: 1, tibionavicular; 2, the tibiospring; 3, tibiocalcaneal; 4, superficial posterior tibiotalar. (*D*) Cadeveric specimen showing the components of the deep deltoid: 5, deep anterior tibiotalar; 6, deep posterior tibiotalar. (*From* Coughlin MJ, Saltzman CL, Anderson RB. Mann's Surgery of the Foot and Ankle, 9th Ed. 2014 Elsevier, Philadelphia, PA; with permission.)

The deep deltoid is the primary restraint to posterior and lateral translation of the talus, in addition to valgus angulation. In contrast, the superficial deltoid resists external rotation of the talus, as well as valgus angulation.[6,7,11]

In rotational ankle fractures (Lauge-Hansen supination external rotation [SER] and PER type injuries[12]), the deltoid may be injured as a result of external rotation. The deltoid may be partially injured or completely ruptured.[13–15] An MRI study of ankle fractures by Jeong and colleagues[14] found that 58% had combined superficial and deep deltoid injuries; 16.7% had superficial only, and 11.1% had deep only. Most superficial and deep anterior deltoid injuries occur proximally at the attachment to the medial malleolus, whereas deep posterior deltoid injuries often occur at the talar insertion.[13–15]

HISTORY OF DELTOID REPAIR

Several authors from the 1960s through the 1990s recommended against repairing the deltoid.[16–22] Most of these studies were based on small case series. In a randomized study of Wb B and C ankle fractures in which the patients underwent fibula fixation with or without suture of the deltoid ligament, Stromsoe and colleagues[18] found no difference in outcomes at a mean of 17 months and recommended against repair of the deltoid. Baird reported on a group of 24 patients, in whom 3 underwent deltoid repair and reported "the three patients with repair did not do as well."[16] On the contrary, Johnson and Hill reported their results treating ankle fractures without deltoid repair and found that, although fixation of the fibula prevented lateral shift and the ankles were considered stable, 41% had fair or poor results, and most had pain medially over the deltoid.[3]

EVALUATION OF THE DELTOID

In the SER ankle fractures, it is imperative to determine stability of the fracture. In the SER II ankle fracture, the fibula is fractured, but the deltoid ligament remains intact, providing a stable ankle mortise. An SER IV equivalent fracture consists of a fibula fracture with injury to the medial structures that leaves the ankle mortise unstable and requires surgical treatment. Although physical examination is critical to evaluation of any injury, it has been shown that medial tenderness is neither sensitive nor specific for identifying deltoid incompetence.[23]

Several studies have shown that gravity and manual external rotation stress radiographs are effective for determining instability in these injuries, with a threshold of greater than 4 mm medial clear space (MCS) as a cutoff for determining instability.[24–27] Rosa and colleagues[28] compared ultrasound to stress radiographs in patients with fibula fractures and found that those patients with an intact deltoid had MCS of 2.7 mm; those with partial tear had 5.2 mm, and those with complete tear had 5.8 mm, with high sensitivity and specificity of ultrasound for diagnosing tears.

MRI has also been shown to be extremely accurate in diagnosing deltoid injuries.[14,29–32] Warner and colleagues[31] found that in cases where the MCS was less than 5 mm on initial (nonstress) injury films, that MRI was more accurate than stress radiography for determining deltoid ligament ruptures; specifically there were more false positives using stress radiographs. They recommended MRI evaluation in patients with initial injury radiographs with MCS less than 5 mm as opposed to stress radiographs. On the contrary, Nortunen and colleagues[30] found a high rate of deltoid ligament disruption in patients with MCS less than 5 mm on stress examination and therefore recommended against obtaining MRI in evaluation of SER IV equivalent ankle fractures. In another study examining MRI findings in patients with Wb B fibula fractures, Lee and colleagues[32] found significantly higher grades of injury in the anterior portion of the deltoid ligament complex in what they considered to be "high-grade unstable fractures," which were those that had residual valgus instability after fibular fixation. There was no difference in the MRI findings of deep deltoid ligament injuries between stable, low-grade unstable, or high-grade unstable fractures. They recommended a grading system based on MRI (**Fig. 2**), which had previously been described by Jeong and colleagues[14]:

- Grade 0 – no damage
- Grade I – periligament edema present
- Grade II – partial tear presenting with laxity, irregular contour or partial discontinuity with hyperintensity of the ligament
- Grade III – complete ligament disruption

RATIONALE FOR REPAIR OF THE DELTOID LIGAMENT

Despite the suggestions that good outcomes may be obtained by repairing the fibula and treating the medial-sided injury nonoperatively, many patients with ankle fractures are not able to return to high levels of athletic activity.[33] It has been shown that lateral talar shift of greater than 2 mm may lead to osteoarthritis of the tibiotalar joint.[34] Additionally, more attention has been paid recently to disability associated with medial ankle instability, and several studies have reported on repair of the deltoid ligament with good outcomes. Hintermann, in a study of 51 patients with medial instability, found surgical repair led to good or excellent results in 90% of patients.[35] In many unstable ankle fractures, the superficial deltoid is completely avulsed off of the medial malleolus, and often interposed in the medial gutter, blocking anatomic reduction of the ankle.[13]

Several studies have reported specifically on the outcomes following deltoid repair in patients with ankle fractures.[13,36–41] Zhao and colleagues[40] reported on retrospective results comparing patients who underwent deltoid repair and those who did not. At a mean follow-up of 53.7 months, they found that the malreduction rate in the non-repair group was 20.4%, with no malreductions in the repair group. Shen and colleagues[37] reported on radiographic and clinical outcomes following suture anchor repair of the deltoid ligament. They found excellent maintenance of the MCS and satisfactory clinical outcomes. Similarly, Ye and colleagues[39] published results from retrospective multicenter study of 131 patients who underwent primary deltoid repair with fibula fracture fixation, and found that no patients developed an increase in MCS or valgus tilt at final follow-up. To the author's knowledge, there are no published prospective randomized controlled trials examining outcomes of deltoid ligament repair in ankle fracture patients.

Despite studies showing satisfactory outcomes after repair of the deltoid ligament in ankle fractures, there is no standard indication to do so. In cases where the fibula is anatomically reduced and the syndesmosis is stable, there should not be lateral translation of the talus with stress. However, there may still be valgus instability or external rotation instability. The author's preferred management strategy is to explore and repair the deltoid ligament in several circumstances:

Patients with frank dislocation or significant MCS widening on stress radiographs
Cases in which the reduction of the talus is prevented by interposed tissue
Cases in which external rotation or valgus instability is still present after anatomic fibula fixation
Cases in which complete deltoid rupture is confirmed arthroscopically

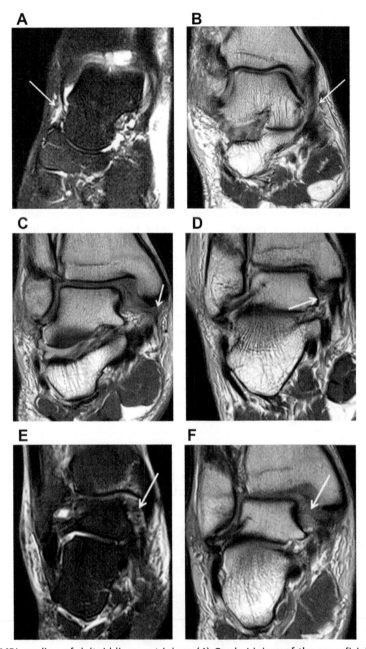

Fig. 2. MRI grading of deltoid ligament injury. (*A*) Grade I injury of the superficial deltoid ligament. (*B*) Grade II injury of the superficial deltoid ligament. (*C*) Grade III injury of the superficial deltoid ligament. (*D*) Grade I injury of the deep posterior deltoid ligament. (*E*) Grade II injury of the deep posterior deltoid ligament. (*F*) Grade III injury of the deep posterior deltoid ligament.[1] (*From* Jeong MS, Choi YS, Kim YJ, Kim JS, Young KW, Jung YY. Deltoid ligament in acute ankle injury: MR imaging analysis. Skeletal Radiol. 2014;43(5):655-663; with permission.)

SURGICAL TECHNIQUE

The fibula fracture is approached initially and prepared for fixation. In cases where a deltoid ligament repair is planned prior, or if proper reduction of the talus is not possible because of interposed soft tissue medially, the approach to the medial ankle is made prior to fixation of the fibula. This allows for greater access to the medial structures and medial ankle joint. A 4 to 5 cm medial incision is made over the medial malleolus extending inferiorly and anteriorly over the deltoid and the posterior tibial tendon sheath. Often a complete avulsion of the superficial deltoid is immediately encountered (**Fig. 3**). The posterior tibial tendon may be retracted inferiorly and posteriorly to expose the deep deltoid insertion on the talus when necessary. The medial aspect of the ankle joint is inspected for loose bodies, and the medial talar dome is inspected for osteochondral injury. The joint is irrigated.

Most commonly, only the superior deltoid avulsion from the medial malleolus is repaired. The anterior aspect of the medial malleolus is roughened with a curette. Two suture anchors are placed In the anterior medial malleolus, approximately 5 mm medial to the articular surface (**Fig. 4**). If the fibula (and if necessary, the syndesmosis) has not been stabilized, it is anatomically reduced and stabilized at this time, prior to final repair of the deltoid. Nonabsorbable sutures from the anchors are then placed in a mattress fashion in the superficial deltoid and secured with the foot and ankle held in a position of internal rotation and inversion. This repair, as well as the anteromedial capsular disruption, is then reinforced with absorbable sutures. The ankle is taken through a range of motion and stressed in external rotation and valgus/eversion to ensure stability.

It is much less common to repair the deep deltoid. As described previously, in cases of deep deltoid rupture, it is most often an avulsion of the distal ligament from the medial talus.[14] If necessary, this may be repaired using 1 or 2 suture anchors placed into the medial talus with nonabsorbable sutures placed in a mattress fashion through the fibers of the deep anterior and posterior deltoid.

ARTHROSCOPY IN ANKLE FRACTURES

Intra-articular pathology has been shown to occur in up to 79% of ankle fractures.[4,42–45] In addition to identifying intra-articular pathology, arthroscopy may allow

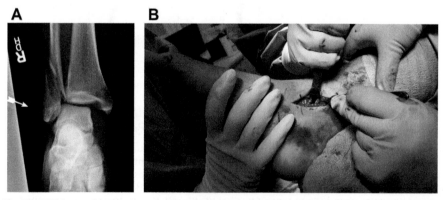

Fig. 3. A 22-year-old man sustained an SER IV equivalent injury while skateboarding. (*A*) Anterior-posterior radiograph without stress demonstrating a fibula fracture with obvious medial clear space widening. (*B*) Intraoperative photograph depicting complete avulsion of the superficial deltoid from the anterior medial malleolus.

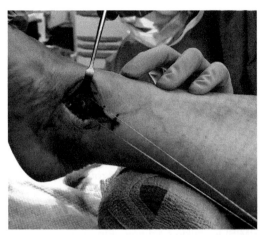

Fig. 4. Intraoperative photo demonstrating the placement of 2 suture anchors in the anterior portion of the medial malleolus used to reattach a complete avulsion of the superficial deltoid to the medial malleolus.

treatment of such injuries, as well as in assuring appropriate reduction of the fractures and syndesmosis instability.

INTRA-ARTICULAR PATHOLOGY

In 2000, Hintermann and colleagues[42] published the results of 288 patients with ankle fractures who underwent arthroscopy at the time of fixation. They found that 79.2% of patients had articular cartilage lesions, with most of these located on the talus. The incidence increased significantly in Wb C type fractures. In addition to the articular cartilage injury, they also found that 14.2% of patients underwent removal of debris, frayed cartilage, or bone fragments arthroscopically. The findings of higher incidence of chondral lesions in patients with Wb C fractures, pronation-external rotation injuries, or syndesmotic injuries has been similarly found by others also.[4,44]

Despite the consistent reports on intra-articular pathology, there are few studies that examine outcomes or the benefit of arthroscopy at the time of ankle fracture surgery. Thordarson and colleagues performed a small prospective randomized trial examining the treatment of trimalleolar fractures with or without arthroscopy. Despite the fact that 8 of 9 patients in the arthroscopy group were found to have articular damage, they did not find any difference in outcomes between the 2 groups.[46] Takao and colleagues[45] performed a prospective study comparing open reduction and internal fixation (ORIF) to arthroscopically assisted ORIF (AAORIF). For articular lesions grades III or IV, they performed drilling of the lesions. At 3.5 years follow-up, they found higher AOFAS scores in the arthroscopy group (91.0) than the ORIF group (87.6). Turhan and colleagues[47] found similar results comparing AAORIF to ORIF in 47 patients with medial malleolar fractures. In their retrospective series of ankle fracture patients treated with ORIF and arthroscopy, Da Cunha and colleagues[44] found that patients with chondral lesions had significantly worse clinical outcomes than those without them; however, they did not have a control group. They also treated lesions with a variety of different techniques and were unable to find a difference in outcomes between them. None of these studies have reported on the actual rate of healing of osteochondral lesions treated at the time of fracture surgery. As reported by Gonzalez and colleagues[48] in a systematic review, arthroscopy may be helpful to identify and treat intra-articular lesions in ankle fractures; however, there is insufficient evidence to identify true benefits in outcomes, and further prospective studies are needed.

In addition to treating articular cartilage lesions, it has been suggested that arthroscopy at the time of ankle fracture fixation may allow for improved detection and treatment of syndesmotic instability.[45,49–52] In a cadaveric model, it was found that arthroscopy had a high sensitivity of detecting sagittal and external rotation instability of the syndesmosis early in the injury pattern, and with low forces applied.[49] Lui and colleagues[51] found that more than twice as many patients with Wb B or C type fractures had syndesmotic instability detected arthroscopically (66%) compared with stress fluoroscopy (30.2%) and concluded that arthroscopy allows better determination of instability in multiple planes (sagittal and rotational) than fluoroscopy alone.

Lastly, as minimally invasive surgical techniques have become more popular in orthopedic surgery, arthroscopy may play a role in furthering this. Chiang and colleagues[52] have described an algorithm for arthroscopic reduction and minimally invasive surgery (ARMIS) for ankle fractures. (**Fig. 5**) They compared this technique to traditional ORIF in 105 patients with SER type ankle fractures. Their technique consists of closed reduction and minimally invasive fixation of the lateral malleolus fracture, ankle arthroscopy for evaluation of syndesmotic injuries, and arthroscopic reduction and percutaneous screw fixation for medial malleolar fractures or detection of deltoid injuries. Although the ARMIS group had longer surgical times, there were fewer complications and reoperations and lower postoperative pain scores. There were no differences in radiographic or functional outcomes.

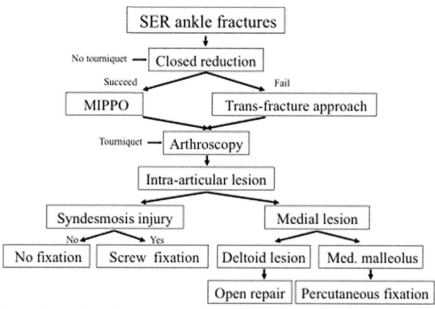

Fig. 5. Algorithm for arthroscopic reduction and minimally invasive surgery (ARMIS) as proposed by Chiang and colleagues (Med, medial; MIPPO, minimally invasive percutaneous plate osteosynthesis; SER, supination-external rotation). (*From* Chiang CC, Tzeng YH, Jeff Lin CF, Wang CS, Lin CC, Chang MC. Arthroscopic Reduction and Minimally Invasive Surgery in Supination-External Rotation Ankle Fractures: A Comparative Study With Open Reduction. *Arthroscopy.* 2019;35(9):2671-2683; with permission.)

SUMMARY

Ankle fractures are extremely common injuries. Recent advances in the understanding of the function of the deltoid ligament complex have led to increased interest in addressing deltoid pathology in conjunction with standard fracture fixation. The aims of repairing the deltoid ligament injury are to improve stability of the ankle joints, specifically in valgus and external rotation, as well as to decrease residual medial pain, which has been found to commonly occur. Additionally, intra-articular pathologies, such as osteochondral lesions, have been found in a high percentage of patients with unstable ankle fractures. Arthroscopy allows for detection and treatment of these lesions, as well as improved detection and treatment of residual instability, specifically of the syndesmosis. However, further prospective studies are needed in both of these areas to further identify which patients will benefit from these additional procedures.

DISCLOSURE

The authors have nothing to disclose.

REFERENCES

1. Court-Brown CM, Caesar B. Epidemiology of adult fractures: A review. Injury 2006;37(8):691–7.
2. Daly PJ, Fitzgerald RH Jr, Melton LJ, et al. Epidemiology of ankle fractures in Rochester, Minnesota. Acta Orthop Scand 1987;58(5):539–44.
3. Johnson DP, Hill J. Fracture-dislocation of the ankle with rupture of the deltoid ligament. Injury 1988;19(2):59–61.
4. Loren GJ, Ferkel RD. Arthroscopic assessment of occult intra-articular injury in acute ankle fractures. Arthroscopy 2002;18(4):412–21.
5. Hintermann B, Knupp M, Pagenstert GI. Deltoid ligament injuries: diagnosis and management. Foot Ankle Clin 2006;11(3):625–37.
6. Rasmussen O, Kromann-Andersen C, Boe S. Deltoid ligament. Functional analysis of the medial collateral ligamentous apparatus of the ankle joint. Acta Orthop Scand 1983;54(1):36–44.
7. Campbell KJ, Michalski MP, Wilson KJ, et al. The ligament anatomy of the deltoid complex of the ankle: a qualitative and quantitative anatomical study. J Bone Joint Surg Am 2014;96(8):e62.
8. Mengiardi B, Pinto C, Zanetti M. Medial collateral ligament complex of the ankle: MR imaging anatomy and findings in medial instability. Semin Musculoskelet Radiol 2016;20(1):91–103.
9. Panchani PN, Chappell TM, Moore GD, et al. Anatomic study of the deltoid ligament of the ankle. Foot Ankle Int 2014;35(9):916–21.
10. Cromeens BP, Kirchhoff CA, Patterson RM, et al. An attachment-based description of the medial collateral and spring ligament complexes. Foot Ankle Int 2015; 36(6):710–21.
11. Harper MC. Deltoid ligament: an anatomical evaluation of function. Foot Ankle 1987;8(1):19–22.
12. Lauge-Hansen N. Fracture of the ankle: II. Combined experimental-surgical and experimental-roentgenologic investigations. Arch Surg 1950;60:957–85.
13. Hsu AR, Lareau CR, Anderson RB. Repair of acute superficial deltoid complex avulsion during ankle fracture fixation in national football league players. Foot Ankle Int 2015;36(11):1272–8.

14. Jeong MS, Choi YS, Kim YJ, et al. Deltoid ligament in acute ankle injury: MR imaging analysis. Skeletal Radiol 2014;43(5):655–63.
15. Mait AR, Forman JL, Nie B, et al. Propagation of Syndesmotic Injuries During Forced External Rotation in Flexed Cadaveric Ankles. Orthop J Sports Med 2018;6(6). 2325967118781333.
16. Baird RA, Jackson ST. Fractures of the distal part of the fibula with associated disruption of the deltoid ligament. Treatment without repair of the deltoid ligament. J Bone Joint Surg Am 1987;69(9):1346–52.
17. Harper MC. The deltoid ligament. An evaluation of need for surgical repair. Clin Orthop Relat Res 1988;(226):156–68.
18. Stromsoe K, Hoqevold HE, Skjeldal S, et al. The repair of a ruptured deltoid ligament is not necessary in ankle fractures. J Bone Joint Surg Br 1995;77(6):920–1.
19. Zeegers AV, van der Werken C. Rupture of the deltoid ligament in ankle fractures: should it be repaired? Injury 1989;20(1):39–41.
20. Bonnin JG. Injury to the ligaments of the ankle. J Bone Joint Surg Br 1965;47(4):609–11.
21. Mast JW, Teipner WA. A reproducible approach to the internal fixation of adult ankle fractures: rationale, technique, and early results. Orthop Clin North Am 1980;11(3):661–79.
22. Yablon IG, Heller FG, Shouse L. The key role of the lateral malleolus in displaced fractures of the ankle. J Bone Joint Surg Am 1977;59(2):169–73.
23. DeAngelis NA, Eskander MS, French BG. Does medial tenderness predict deep deltoid ligament incompetence in supination-external rotation type ankle fractures? J Orthop Trauma 2007;21(4):244–7.
24. Gill JB, Risko T, Raducan V, et al. Comparison of manual and gravity stress radiographs for the evaluation of supination-external rotation fibular fractures. J Bone Joint Surg Am 2007;89(5):994–9.
25. Michelson JD, Varner KE, Checcone M. Diagnosing deltoid injury in ankle fractures: the gravity stress view. Clin Orthop Relat Res 2001;387:178–82.
26. Schock HJ, Pinzur M, Manion L, et al. The use of gravity or manual-stress radiographs in the assessment of supination-external rotation fractures of the ankle. J Bone Joint Surg Br 2007;89(8):1055–9.
27. LeBa TB, Gugala Z, Morris RP, et al. Gravity versus manual external rotation stress view in evaluating ankle stability: a prospective study. Foot Ankle Spec 2015;8(3):175–9.
28. Rosa I, Rodeia J, Fernandes PX, et al. Ultrasonographic assessment of deltoid ligament integrity in ankle fractures. Foot Ankle Int 2019;41(2):147–53.
29. Cheung Y, Perrich KD, Gui J, et al. MRI of isolated distal fibular fractures with widened medial clear space on stressed radiographs: which ligaments are interrupted? AJR Am J Roentgenol 2009;192(1):W7–12.
30. Nortunen S, Lepojarvi S, Savola O, et al. Stability assessment of the ankle mortise in supination-external rotation-type ankle fractures: lack of additional diagnostic value of MRI. J Bone Joint Surg Am 2014;96(22):1855–62.
31. Warner SJ, Garner MR, Fabricant PD, et al. The diagnostic accuracy of radiographs and magnetic resonance imaging in predicting deltoid ligament ruptures in ankle fractures. HSS J 2019;15(2):115–21.
32. Lee TH, Jang KS, Choi GW, et al. The contribution of anterior deltoid ligament to ankle stability in isolated lateral malleolar fractures. Injury 2016;47(7):1581–5.
33. Hong CC, Roy SP, Nashi N, et al. Functional outcome and limitation of sporting activities after bimalleolar and trimalleolar ankle fractures. Foot Ankle Int 2013;34(6):805–10.

34. Harris J, Fallat L. Effects of isolated Weber B fibular fractures on the tibiotalar contact area. J Foot Ankle Surg 2004;43(1):3–9.
35. Hintermann B, Valderrabano V, Boss A, et al. Medial ankle instability: an exploratory, prospective study of fifty-two cases. Am J Sports Med 2004;32(1):183–90.
36. Jones CR, Nunley JA 2nd. Deltoid ligament repair versus syndesmotic fixation in bimalleolar equivalent ankle fractures. J Orthop Trauma 2015;29(5):245–9.
37. Shen JJ, Gao YB, Huang JF, et al. Suture anchors for primary deltoid ligament repair associated with acute ankle fractures. Acta Orthop Belg 2019;85(3):387–91.
38. Wang X, Zhang C, Yin JW, et al. Treatment of medial malleolus or pure deltoid ligament injury in patients with supination-external rotation type IV ankle fractures. Orthop Surg 2017;9(1):42–8.
39. Yu GR, Zhang MZ, Aiyer A, et al. Repair of the acute deltoid ligament complex rupture associated with ankle fractures: a multicenter clinical study. J Foot Ankle Surg 2015;54(2):198–202.
40. Zhao HM, Lu J, Zhang F, et al. Surgical treatment of ankle fracture with or without deltoid ligament repair: a comparative study. BMC Musculoskelet Disord 2017;18(1):543.
41. Woo SH, Bae SY, Chung HJ. Short-term results of a ruptured deltoid ligament repair during an acute ankle fracture fixation. Foot Ankle Int 2018;39(1):35–45.
42. Hintermann B, Regazzoni P, Lampert C, et al. Arthroscopic findings in acute fractures of the ankle. J Bone Joint Surg Br 2000;82(3):345–51.
43. Leontaritis N, Hinojosa L, Panchbhavi VK. Arthroscopically detected intra-articular lesions associated with acute ankle fractures. J Bone Joint Surg Am 2009;91(2):333–9.
44. Da Cunha RJ, Karnovsky SC, Schairer W, et al. Ankle arthroscopy for diagnosis of full-thickness talar cartilage lesions in the setting of acute ankle fractures. Arthroscopy 2018;34(6):1950–7.
45. Takao M, Uchio Y, Naito K, et al. Diagnosis and treatment of combined intra-articular disorders in acute distal fibular fractures. J Trauma 2004;57(6):1303–7.
46. Thordarson DB, Bains R, Shepherd LE. The role of ankle arthroscopy on the surgical management of ankle fractures. Foot Ankle Int 2001;22(2):123–5.
47. Turhan E, Doral MN, Demirel M, et al. Arthroscopy-assisted reduction versus open reduction in the fixation of medial malleolar fractures. Eur J Orthop Surg Traumatol 2013;23(8):953–9.
48. Gonzalez TA, Macaulay AA, Ehrlichman LK, et al. Arthroscopically assisted versus standard open reduction and internal fixation techniques for the acute ankle fracture. Foot Ankle Int 2016;37(5):554–62.
49. Watson BC, Lucas DE, Simpson GA, et al. Arthroscopic evaluation of syndesmotic instability in a cadaveric model. Foot Ankle Int 2015;36(11):1362–8.
50. Chan KB, Lui TH. Role of ankle arthroscopy in management of acute ankle fracture. Arthroscopy 2016;32(11):2373–80.
51. Lui TH, Ip K, Chow HT. Comparison of radiologic and arthroscopic diagnoses of distal tibiofibular syndesmosis disruption in acute ankle fracture. Arthroscopy 2005;21(11):1370.
52. Chiang CC, Tzeng YH, Jeff Lin CF, et al. Arthroscopic reduction and minimally invasive surgery in supination-external rotation ankle fractures: a comparative study with open reduction. Arthroscopy 2019;35(9):2671–83.

Acute and Chronic Syndesmotic Instability
Role of Surgical Stabilization

Derek S. Stenquist, MD[a],*, Michael Y. Ye, BSE[b],
John Y. Kwon, MD[b]

KEYWORDS

- Syndesmosis • Tibiofibular • Instability • High ankle sprain

KEY POINTS

- Acute or chronic syndesmotic injuries can significantly impact athletic function and activities of daily living.
- Patient history, examination, and the judicious use of imaging modalities aid diagnosis. Surgical management should be used when frank diastasis, instability, and/or chronic pain and disability ensue.
- Screw and suture-button fixation remain the mainstay of treatment of acute injuries, but novel syndesmotic reconstruction techniques hold promise for treatment of acute and chronic injuries, especially for athletes.

INTRODUCTION

Ankle fractures account for more than 50% of lower extremity fractures and 14% of fracture-related hospital admissions.[1,2] Approximately 20% occur with concomitant syndesmotic injury.[3,4] In athletic populations, syndesmotic injuries account for up to 25% of ankle sprains.[5–7] Approximately 6500 syndesmotic injuries occur yearly in the United States based on emergency room admissions data.[8] Syndesmotic injuries have demonstrated increased recovery times[9,10] and have the potential to cause long-term disability.[10] They are 30% more common in men and most occur in adults aged 18 to 34.[8]

Syndesmotic injury with persistent diastasis or dynamic instability is associated with pain and dysfunction and requires surgical stabilization.[11,12] Malreduction has been shown to be a significant predictor of poor outcomes.[12–14] Symptomatic osteoarthritis can occur within 7 years in 11% of ankle fractures requiring syndesmotic fixation, with malreduction being an independent predictor for its

[a] Harvard Combined Orthopaedic Residency Program, 55 Fruit Street, Boston, MA 02114, USA;
[b] Carl J. Shapiro Department of Orthopaedics, Beth Israel Deaconess Medical Center, 330 Brookline Avenue, Boston, MA 02215, USA
* Corresponding author.
E-mail address: dstenquist@mgh.harvard.edu

Clin Sports Med 39 (2020) 745–771
https://doi.org/10.1016/j.csm.2020.06.002
0278-5919/20/© 2020 Elsevier Inc. All rights reserved.

development.[15] Because syndesmotic injuries occur most commonly in young adults, proper diagnosis and treatment is necessary to allow for return to athletic activities and to avoid long-term sequela.

In this review, we focus on anatomy, mechanisms of injury, diagnosis, and surgical reduction and stabilization of acute and chronic syndesmotic instability. We discuss various fixation methods with a focus on considerations for the athlete.

ANATOMY

The distal tibiofibular syndesmosis maintains the relationship between the tibia and fibula to stabilize the talocrural joint.[16] The distal tibiofibular syndesmosis is comprised of two bones and four connecting structures: the anterior inferior tibiofibular ligament (AITFL), posterior inferior tibiofibular ligament (PITFL), interosseous ligament (IOL), and interosseous membrane (IOM).[16]

Bony Anatomy

The syndesmosis consists of a triangular tibial groove called the incisura tibialis that articulates with the distal fibula. The proximal apex begins where the lateral tibial ridge bifurcates forming anterior and posterior margins that terminate distally as Chaput and Volkmann tubercle, respectively.[16] This bifurcation occurs approximately 6 to 8 cm proximal to the plafond. A corresponding bifurcation of the fibula matches the concave shape of the incisura tibialis. Significant anatomic variation exists with varying osseous morphology,[16] which may potentially predispose to injury and risk of malreduction.[16,17] Chaput tubercle is generally more prominent than Volkmann tubercle and overlaps the medial two-thirds of the anterior distal fibula.[16] The anterior fibular tubercle (Wagstaffe-Le Fort tubercle) is more prominent than the posterior fibular tubercle.[16,18]

Tibiofibular Contact Area/Syndesmotic Recess

This articulation between the distal tibia and fibula is the tibiofibular contact area, which varies in size from 3 to 9 mm anterior to posterior and 2 to 5 mm in height.[7,16] Although Bartonicek[19] found this articulation to be variably present, Williams and colleagues[7] noted articulating cartilage facets in 100% of cadavers examined. The articular facets may provide landmarks for restoration of syndesmotic alignment.[16,19] The syndesmotic recess is a synovial joint or plica, which is contiguous with the tibiotalar joint and bordered anteriorly by the AITFL and superiorly by the IOM (**Fig. 1**).[7,19] Contrast leakage proximal to this synovial cavity during arthrogram performed for suspected injury may indicate acute AITFL tear.[16]

Anterior Inferior Tibiofibular Ligament

The AITFL consists of three to five bands and runs distolaterally from the tibia to the fibula.[7] The bands converge distally giving it a trapezoidal shape (**Fig. 2**).[7,16] An anomalous distal fascicle can exist termed the Bassett ligament. Bassett ligament can cause symptomatic ankle impingement and is resected without causing instability.[16] The AITFL contributes approximately 35% of the strength of the syndesmosis,[20] and is likely the first to yield with supraphysiologic external rotation (ER).[16]

Posterior Inferior Tibiofibular Ligament

The PITFL also runs distolaterally from the tibia to the fibula (**Fig. 3**). It has superficial and deep components, and together they contribute approximately 42% of the strength of the syndesmosis.[20] The superficial PITFL is trapezoidal with multiple

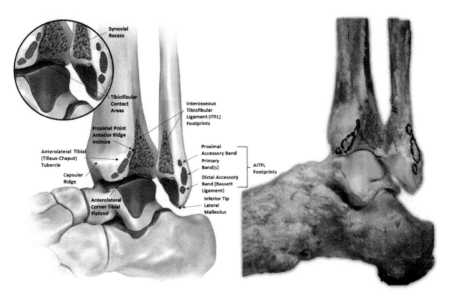

Fig. 1. Anterolateral "open book" view of the left ankle with the fibula externally rotated to demonstrate the IOL.[7] The tibiofibular contact area is an articulation between the distal tibia and fibula. The articular facets may provide landmarks for restoration of syndesmotic alignment. The syndesmotic recess is a synovial joint or plica that is contiguous with the tibiotalar joint (*inset*). (*From* Williams BT, Ahrberg AB, Goldsmith MT, et al. Ankle syndesmosis: a qualitative and quantitative anatomic analysis. Am J Sports Med. 2015;43(1):88-97; with permission.)

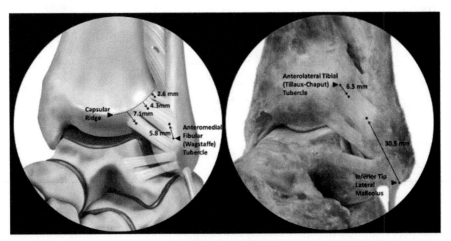

Fig. 2. Anterolateral view of the left ankle. The AITFL originates approximately 9 mm superior to the anterolateral corner of the tibial plafond and inserts approximately 30 mm superior to the tip of the lateral malleolus. From proximal to distal, proximal accessory band, primary band, Bassett ligament.[7] (*From* Williams BT, Ahrberg AB, Goldsmith MT, et al. Ankle syndesmosis: a qualitative and quantitative anatomic analysis. Am J Sports Med. 2015;43(1):88-97; with permission.)

fascicles converging distally.[7] The deep PITFL (also known as the inferior transverse ligament) has more dense fibers and a thicker, rounder shape.[7,16] The PITFL has a broad origin on Volkmann tubercle, which forms part of the posterior malleolus. Ligamentous strength often results in a bony tubercle avulsion rather than pure ligamentous rupture with rotational injuries.[16] Although posterior malleolus fracture morphology can vary,[21] the PITFL often remains intact according to MRI studies.[22] The PITFL's osseous attachments have important implications for posterior malleolar fixation affecting stability,[23] syndesmotic reduction,[22] and functional outcomes[24] after ankle fractures.

Interosseous Ligament

The IOL originates at the distal margin of the IOM. Most of its fibers run distolaterally from the tibia.[7] Its tibial origin is approximately 5 cm proximal to the tibial plafond and its fibular origin 7 cm proximal to the tip of the lateral malleolus.[7,16] Biomechanical studies have found that the IOL contributes up to 22% of the strength of the syndesmosis.[20] It is thought to function as a spring between the tibia and fibula allowing the

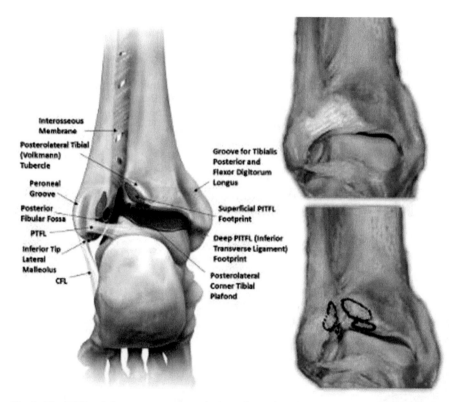

Fig. 3. The PITFL originates approximately 8 cm from the posterolateral corner of the tibial plafond and runs distally and laterally to its insertion on the fibula approximately 26 mm superior to the tip of the lateral malleolus.[7] The deep PITFL originates 8 mm distal to the superficial PITFL on the tibia, running horizontally to insert on the posterior fibula.[7,16] CFL, calcaneofibular ligament. (*From* Williams BT, Ahrberg AB, Goldsmith MT, et al. Ankle syndesmosis: a qualitative and quantitative anatomic analysis. Am J Sports Med. 2015;43(1):88-97; with permission.)

talus to wedge in the mortise during dorsiflexion and neutralizing forces during stance phase.[16]

Interosseous Membrane

The IOM runs between the lateral tibial ridge and the medial fibular ridge. It terminates as the IOL, a transition, which occurs approximately at the bifurcation of the tibial ridge to form the incisura tibialis. Like the IOL, the IOM also seems to be loaded throughout stance phase.[16] Although the IOM contributes to syndesmotic stability, it plays a minor role compared with other components.[20] McKeon and colleagues[25] performed a cadaver study to elucidate the vascular supply of the syndesmosis, which showed that the syndesmotic branch of the peroneal artery supplying the anterior syndesmosis may be at risk when syndesmotic injury extends into the IOM (**Fig. 4**).

Deltoid Ligament

The deltoid ligament (DL), although not strictly part of the syndesmosis, contributes directly to mortise stability acting as a tether against lateral talar translation and rotation.[9] There is a high rate of concomitant injury with approximately 50% of patients with DL disruption having an associated syndesmotic injury.[26] In a cadaveric study, Massri-Pugin and colleagues[27] found that isolated DL disruption or sectioning of the DL and AITFL did not render the syndesmosis unstable to lateral hook testing.

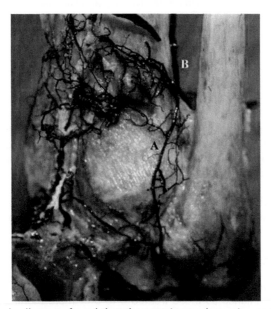

Fig. 4. McKeon and colleagues found that the anterior syndesmosis was supplied primarily by a perforating branch (A) of the peroneal artery (B) in two-thirds of cadaveric specimens, with supplemental perfusion from branches of the anterior tibial artery approximately one-third of the time. The syndesmotic branch of the peroneal artery perforates the IOM approximately 3 cm proximal to the tibiotalar joint, placing the blood supply to the anterior syndesmosis at risk when injury extends into the IOM. The posterior syndesmosis was supplied primarily by a posterior branch of the peroneal artery with additional contributions from branches of the posterior tibial artery in approximately one-third of cadavers. (*From* McKeon KE, Wright RW, Johnson JE, McCormick JJ KS. Vascular anatomy of the tibiofibular syndesmosis. J Bone Jt Surg Am. 2012;94:931-938; with permission.)

However, the syndesmosis became unstable if the DL was disrupted in combination with the AITFL and IOL. In another study[28] the same group demonstrated that isolated disruption of the AITFL and IOL was not enough to produce coronal instability. Therefore, concomitant DL disruption may produce instability even with an intact PITFL.[27] Using computed tomography (CT) scans of cadaveric ankles to study talar kinematics under stress testing, Goetz and colleagues[29] demonstrated significant differences between instability patterns in the intact state, with isolated deep DL disruption, and with disruption of the DL and syndesmotic ligaments. This further demonstrates the DL's role in mortise stability. Surgeons must have a high suspicion for instability in injuries to the syndesmosis that also involve the DL.[27]

MECHANISM OF INJURY

Mechanism of injury involves forceful ER of the dorsiflexed foot.[9,30] Lauge-Hansen's mechanistic theory postulated that the pronated foot position puts the DL on tension, thus initially creating a medial-sided injury. As an ER force is applied through the ankle, the AITFL is disrupted followed closely by the posterior elements. As the rotational force continues, a high fibula fracture occurs with the resultant fracture pattern determined by the predominant deforming force (ER vs abduction).[3,27] Although occurring in approximately 20% of supination-external injuries, there is a higher incidence of syndesmotic injury with pronation-type injuries.[31] Syndesmotic injuries commonly occur during contact sports, which involve lateral movements and may be related to external foot constraint.[9,10,32]

CLASSIFICATION

Classification systems are based on symptomatology and associated instability determined largely by radiographic findings. There have been several classifications[10,33–35] described, albeit of limited clinical utility. A simple grading system has been most commonly used.[9,36] Grade I injuries demonstrate a stable syndesmosis with mild symptoms and normal radiographic findings indicating ligamentous sprain. Although stability of grade II injuries is debated, they are considered to have partial syndesmotic complex disruption. Clinical tests may be positive but radiographic findings are normal. The DL status becomes important to stability when the AITFL and IOL are disrupted. Therefore, some authors consider concomitant DL disruption on MRI as an indication for surgical stabilization in the setting of a grade II injury.[36] In grade III injuries, the AITFL, PITFL, IOL, and DL are disrupted with clear malalignment on plain radiographs requiring operative stabilization.[9,36]

ACUTE AND CHRONIC INJURY

Many authors have defined acute injuries as those treated within 1 to 3 months of injury and chronic injuries as those treated 3 to 6 or more months after injury.[37–39] Acute syndesmotic injury should be suspected after any rotational ankle injury[9] because up to 15% of ankle sprains in National Collegiate Athletic Association athletes are syndesmotic sprains.[32] Indications for nonoperative management of acute injury include grade I or II injuries without clinical ankle instability or radiographic diastasis.[9] Typically with isolated injury to the AITFL or DL, nonoperative management with a short period of immobilization followed by functional rehabilitation is recommended.[9] For stable acute injuries, athletes can expect to return to competition within 2 to 6 weeks,[40] although prolonged healing can occur and persistent pain may warrant further investigation.[9] Acute grade II injuries with dynamic instability and grade III injuries are managed surgically. The mean time to return to full sporting activity after surgical management is approximately 9 to 10 weeks for professional athletes.[41,42] Clinical determination of instability is difficult because tests for syndesmotic instability are of limited reliability.[9,30] During attempted nonoperative management of acute syndesmotic injuries, a high index of suspicion for instability and close follow-up are essential to prevent time lost from sport or progression to chronic injury.

Despite the lack of consensus regarding definition, treatment of subacute and chronic syndesmotic injuries is necessarily dictated by the structures injured and the nature of injury. For example, for subacute injuries Van den Bekerom and colleagues[37] recommend restoration of the normal anatomy with screw placement and tendon repair or grafting depending on the adequacy of tendon remnants. For chronic injuries with persistent diastasis, they noted that syndesmotic fusion may be required. Although acute versus chronic syndesmotic injuries are technically defined by chronicity, treatment is dictated by the constellation of symptomatology, clinical examination, radiographic and advanced imaging findings, and functional demands of the patient. In this context, the diagnosis of syndesmotic pathology is discussed next followed by various options for surgical management.

DIAGNOSIS

Syndesmotic injuries are difficult to diagnose regardless of mechanism or associated injuries because of a lack of consensus on criteria and variable reliability of diagnostic tests.[30] The role of different imaging modalities and stress examination is also debated.[43,44]

History

Although some patients may recall an eversion or forceful ER,[30] they are often unable to recount a definite mechanism, unlike patients sustaining simple inversion injuries.[36] Symptoms may include pain above the ankle joint, subjective instability, or a history of protracted recovery.[36] The history for chronic syndesmotic injury is often more subtle and patients may complain of a sensation of giving way, difficulty with walking on uneven ground, ankle stiffness, or limited dorsiflexion.[37] Some patients exhibit chronic dynamic syndesmotic instability in the form of persistent symptoms without objective radiographic diastasis, also known as functional instability, making diagnosis difficult.[37]

Physical Examination

Patients classically have tenderness above the ankle joint at the level of the AITFL. They may have tenderness with palpation of the posterior syndesmosis and associated swelling.[30,36] Several clinical tests have been described, albeit with variable sensitivity, specificity, and reliability.[30,36] The ER stress test is performed by externally rotating the foot with the knee at 90° and the ankle in neutral. Pain over the syndesmosis is a positive result. The dorsiflexion range of motion test involves passive ankle dorsiflexion with a positive test demonstrating reduced motion secondary to pain inhibition compared with the contralateral ankle. The dorsiflexion with compression test has the patient actively dorsiflex with the examiner compressing the malleoli. Either an increase in ankle dorsiflexion or decrease in pain with compression constitutes a positive test. The "squeeze test" is positive when proximal compression of the tibia and fibula causes pain distally at the syndesmosis. In a systematic review, Sman and colleagues[30] found low diagnostic accuracy of all these clinical tests. However, a positive squeeze test was associated with longer time lost from competition and may be useful for prognosis. The ER stress test and squeeze test both demonstrated high specificity but low sensitivity when correlated with MRI findings. Furthermore, although interobserver reliability has been demonstrated to be high for the ER stress test, squeeze test, and dorsiflexion range of motion test, it has shown to be moderate to poor for others. Given this, providers should not rely on a single test but should use a combination of history, examination, and imaging findings.[30]

IMAGING
Radiographic Evaluation

Definitive radiographic findings for the diagnosis of syndesmotic injury may be limited except in cases of obvious instability. Although initial descriptions or tibiofibular clear space (TFCS) and tibiofibular overlap (TFO) date back to Lauge-Hansen's works, Harper and Keller[45] more formally established normative data as measured on anteroposterior and mortise radiographs. The utility of these parameters has been investigated for detecting syndesmotic injury and for determining syndesmotic reduction postoperatively. Although TFCS and TFO are important parameters, others have found that asymptomatic patients may meet traditional radiographic thresholds for syndesmotic injury.[36,46] Radiographic comparison with the contralateral ankle may be more useful than using population norms.[36,46] Shah and colleagues[46] determined that the TFCS measured on the mortise view is the most accurate parameter when using a comparison contralateral radiograph. Marmor and colleagues[47] demonstrated the limitations of plain radiographs for detecting syndesmotic malreduction in a cadaver model. When assessing various degrees of rotational malalignment, they demonstrated that up to 30° of ER malalignment can go undetected when using TFCS and TFO.[47] Despite its limitations, radiographs should always be obtained as the initial imaging modality.

Radiographic Stress Testing

Radiographic stress testing, in the form of manual ER or gravity stress, may aid in diagnosis.[9] Intraoperative stress testing after fibular fixation should always be performed to assess syndesmotic integrity.[9] Intraoperative assessment is most commonly performed using a lateral fibular stress test (Cotton test) or ER stress test.[48] The Cotton test is performed by applying a lateral distraction force using a surgical clamp applied to the distal fibula approximately 1 to 2 cm proximal to the plafond. For the ER stress test, the ankle is held in neutral plantarflexion while an ER force is applied to the foot with the tibia stabilized.[48] Regardless of test, medial clear space, TFO, and TFCS should be examined and compared with the contralateral uninjured ankle. Although some authors have suggested the Cotton test to be insufficiently sensitive,[48] other biomechanical studies suggest the ER stress test may in fact overestimate instability.[49] Although stress radiography is a useful adjunct, many factors influence accuracy including ankle position and force applied.[50,51]

Computed Tomography

CT is more sensitive than plain radiography for detecting malalignment, although contralateral imaging is recommended because of variations in population norms.[36,52,53] Multiple authors have examined means of measuring syndesmotic alignment using CT.[52–54] Nault and colleagues[52] established a set of reliable measurements and normative values for syndesmotic alignment using CT scans of 100 normal ankles. Patel and colleagues[55] applied these methods to study a cohort of uninjured patients undergoing bilateral weightbearing CT. They found little side-to-side variation, supporting the use of simultaneous bilateral imaging.[55] Hagemeijer and co-workers[44] studied bilateral weightbearing CT of patients with known syndesmotic instability compared with normal control subjects and found CT effective in diagnosing diastasis. Although the most accurate, reliable, and practical measurement technique has yet to be determined, investigations continue because CT is currently the most sensitive imaging modality for detecting subtle syndesmotic malalignment. Given high rates of syndesmotic disruption and malreduction in ankle fractures, bilateral CT imaging is the modality of choice for postoperative evaluation especially in the setting of metal implants.

MRI

MRI has been shown to have high sensitivity and specificity for detecting acute syndesmotic injury as confirmed by arthroscopy and direct surgical visualization.[43] However, MRI is static and cannot detect dynamic instability.[36] MRI may also be useful for diagnosing chronic disruption.[56] Ryan and colleagues[57] found that a positive "lambda sign" on the coronal view of gadolinium-enhanced MRI, in combination with positive clinical findings, demonstrated 75% sensitivity and 85% specificity for latent injury defined as greater than 2-mm translation on arthroscopic stress examination. Furthermore, MRI may be useful for detection of concomitant injuries, such as lateral ligament injury, peroneal tendon tears, and osteochondral lesions. In the setting of suspicious examination findings and unremarkable plain radiographs, MRI should be considered acutely or for persistent symptomology.

Arthroscopy

Arthroscopy allows surgeons to visualize and measure dynamic diastasis and distinguish instability in multiple planes (**Fig. 5**D).[28,58] Threshold measurements for diagnosing instability continue to evolve.[59] Guyton and colleagues[59] argued that traditional criteria of 2-mm fibular translation in any plane tends to overdiagnose instability. Massri-Pugin and colleagues[28] sequentially disrupted syndesmotic ligaments in 14 cadavers and assessed coronal plane motion. They found that the AITFL, IOL, and PITFL all need to be transected to produce coronal plane diastasis and that arthroscopic assessment of coronal instability is best made along the posterior incisural margin. Coronal diastasis at the anterior incisural margin was associated with additional DL disruption. Lubberts and colleagues[60] demonstrated an increase in sagittal diastasis after sectioning of all three syndesmotic ligaments or with partial transection of the AITFL and IOL in combination with complete DL transection, demonstrating the role of the DL. Based on receiver operating characteristic curve analysis, they concluded that the optimal arthroscopic cutoff point to distinguish a stable from unstable syndesmosis was 2 mm of total fibular translation in the sagittal plane, which yielded a sensitivity of 77.5% and specificity of 88.9%.[60]

ACHIEVING REDUCTION

Reported rates of malreduction after surgical fixation range from 16% to 52%.[61,62] Methods for achieving reduction include clamp placement, manual or "thumb" reduction, or reduction via implant placement.[63] Manual reduction outperformed clamp and screw or suture-button (SB) fixation as measured by restoration of normal joint contact forces in a cadaver study.[36,63] Direct open visualization seems to be superior to indirect reduction. Indirect reduction with a clamp and screw technique has reported malreduction rates of 50%,[64] whereas direct visualization has been found to be 16%.[61] A recent study by Tornetta and colleagues[65] suggested the anterior articular surface to be a

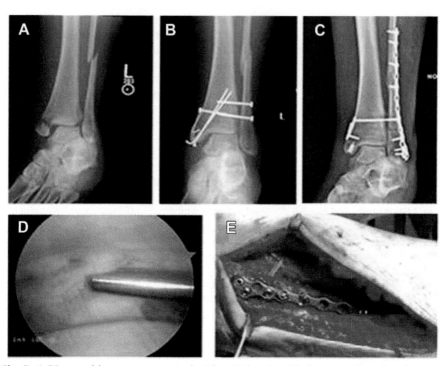

Fig. 5. A 56-year-old woman presented with a Weber C ankle fracture (*A*) and underwent open reduction internal fixation (ORIF) at an outside facility. She presented 9 months postoperatively with complaints of pain and instability and was found to have a fibular malunion with failure of syndesmotic fixation resulting in chronic syndesmotic instability (*B*). Ankle arthroscopy confirmed syndesmotic instability (*D*) and she underwent revision ORIF (*C*) including deltoid ligament repair and syndesmotic reconstruction with an internal brace as described by Regauer and colleagues (*E*).[159] A 2.7-mm bone tunnel is created in the distal fibula between the fibular footprints of the AITFL and PITFL. Suture-tape is then passed through the bone tunnel until the middle of the tape is inside the tunnel and secured with an anchor. After a 3.4-mm bone tunnel is created in the distal tibia between the tibial footprints of the AITFL and PITFL, the free ends of the suture-tape are secured into the tibial bone tunnel.[159]

significantly more accurate visual reference than the incisura for direct open reduction. Specific clamp and screw angles may predispose to malreduction[66,67] and incisural anatomy influences the type of malreduction that can occur (**Fig. 6**B).[17] However, a recent prospective trial demonstrated no difference in functional outcomes between patients treated with clamp versus manual reduction.[68] Although the use of intraoperative three-dimensional CT has been shown to decrease malreduction,[69] this resource is not widely available. An understanding of the pitfalls and predisposing factors for syndesmotic malreduction can help surgeons optimize outcomes.

Screw Fixation

Metal screws have long been used for syndesmotic fixation. Multiple studies have examined the number, location, diameter, and positioning of screws. Although cadaveric studies suggest that larger diameter screws better resist shear stress, under cyclic loading neither diameter demonstrated a biomechanical advantage.[70,71] Markolf and colleagues[72] found no differences in stability with screw size. Stuart and

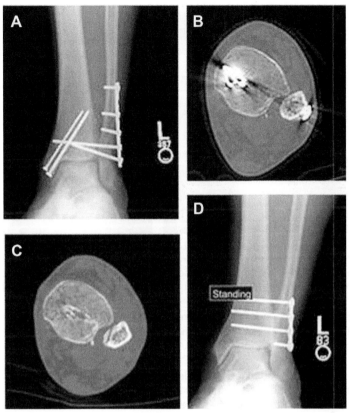

Fig. 6. A 58-year-old man underwent ORIF of a left Weber B ankle fracture at an outside institution (*A*). He presented with persistent pain and was found to have an anterior syndesmotic malreduction (*B*). He failed removal of hardware (*C*) and ultimately required syndesmotic arthrodesis (*D*).

Panchbhavi[73] reported that 3.5-mm screws break more frequently than 4.0- or 4.5-mm screws. Lee and colleagues[74] reported good stability, no breakage, and low risk of complications using 5.0-mm partially threaded cannulated quadricortical screws. An initial study of the R3lease screw (Paragon 28, Englewood, CO), a novel syndesmotic screw with a specific break point, demonstrated good initial short-term results (**Fig. 7**B).[75]

The literature reports conflicting information regarding the suitability of tricortical or quadricortical screw application. Moore and colleagues[76] and Markolf and colleagues[72] reported no difference in stability or outcomes, although Moore noted a trend toward higher loss of reduction with tricortical fixation. Serhan and colleagues[77] reported in a finite element analysis that a single 3.5-mm quadricortical screw experienced the highest stress, whereas a single 4.5-mm quadricortical screw experienced the least. Høiness and Strømsøe found no difference in outcomes between a single quadricortical 4.5-mm screw and two 3.5-mm tricortical screws.[78] Serhan and colleagues[77] reported no difference between the use of either one or two 3.5-mm tricortical screws. A computational biomechanical model by Li and colleagues[79] found that in neutral, externally rotated, and internally rotated positions, a tricortical screw better restored normal articular contact force and experienced less peak stress compared

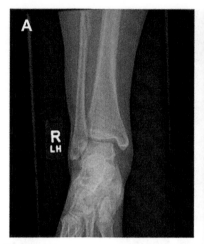
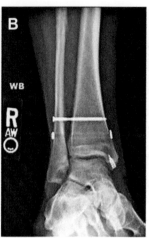

Fig. 7. A 33-year-old woman sustained a Weber C ankle fracture while roller skating (*A*). She underwent ORIF including fixation of the syndesmosis with a combination of controlled break point screw and suture button because of the length and unstable nature of the fibula fracture (*B*). Fixation was augmented with deltoid ligament suture-anchor repair.

with a quadricortical screw. Systematic reviews have concluded that in general, the number of screws, screw diameter, and the number of cortices engaged had no effect on clinical outcomes and no definitive correlation with loss of syndesmotic reduction.[80,81]

Ideal screw trajectory continues to be debated. The Arbeitsgemeinschaft für Osteosynthesefragen Foundation recommends that syndesmotic screws be placed parallel and 2 cm proximal to the plafond and inserted obliquely posterior to anterior at an angle of 25° to 30°.[82] Mendelsohn and colleagues[83] reported that the distal tibiofibular axis is 32 ± 6° externally rotated from the transepicondylar femoral axis. Despite these traditional recommendations, authors have increasingly shown that individual anatomic variation makes finding the ideal clamp position and screw trajectory challenging.[17,84] Regarding screw position relative to the plafond, several authors have found no difference in clinical or radiologic outcomes between trans-syndesmotic and suprasyndesmotic screw placement.[73,85–87] Most clinical studies on this topic suffer from low sample size and larger prospective studies are needed.[80] Currently, it seems that acceptable outcomes are achieved by placing syndesmotic fixation between 2 and 5 cm proximal to the plafond.

Routine screw removal is a historic recommendation and is commonly performed despite limited clinical benefit.[88] In past surveys, most surgeons have reported performing routine screw removal.[89,90] Intact syndesmotic screws restricted physiologic fibular motion in a cadaver model,[91] and Manjoo and colleagues[92] reported worse functional outcomes in patients with intact screws compared with broken, loosened, or removed screws. Screw retention may be of particular concern for athletes, although Briceno and colleagues[93] recently demonstrated no increase in ankle dorsiflexion with screw removal. Recent systematic reviews have recommended against routine screw removal given little demonstrated clinical, radiographic, or functional benefit.[80,94,95] Despite the existing literature, however, screw removal may be considered in the high-level athlete for several reasons: (1) this healthy patient population typically has low surgical and anesthetic risk, (2) nonphysiologic kinematics produced by a retained screw may affect athletes more than others given high functional demands, and (3) current patient-based outcome measures used in previous investigations may have an undefined ceiling effect such that high-level athletes may actually exhibit benefit from screw removal.

Bioabsorbable Screws

An alternative to metal screw fixation is the use of bioabsorbable screws,[96–102] which may negate need for removal and produce a gradual transfer of stress that results in improved healing.[97,103,104] Bioabsorbable screws are typically made of either polyglycolide acid, polylactide acid, polylevolactic acid (PLLA), or copolymers.[102,105,106] Each material has a different degradation rate based on its biochemical properties.[104] PLLA degrades more slowly and retains more strength over time and thus may be more suitable for syndesmotic fixation.[102,104,107] Cadaveric studies have shown that bioabsorbable screws demonstrate near biomechanical equivalence to metal screws of same diameter for syndesmotic fixation.[99,108] Meta-analyses comparing bioabsorbable with metal screws have found similar outcomes and range of motion.[105,106,109] Despite no statistical difference in complication rates, meta-analysis has demonstrated a trend toward higher complications for bioabsorbable screws, especially foreign body reaction.[105,106,109,110] Polyglycolide acid screws in particular have been associated with delayed inflammatory reactions and sterile abscesses,[111–113] leading to general abandonment.[100] PLLA screws have a lower reported incidence of inflammatory reactions.[104,107] Bioabsorbable screws may be a compelling option for syndesmotic fixation in athletes moving forward, but given the lower cost, reliability, availability, and surgeon-familiarity with metal screws or SB devices, bioabsorbable screws continue to have a limited role in current practice.

Suture-Button Fixation

Over the past decade, SB fixation for syndesmotic disruption has grown in popularity (see **Fig. 7B**). A biomechanical study by Pang and colleagues[114] demonstrated that a double SB construct more closely matched the intact state in terms of mortise contact and pressure mechanics with an applied axial load as compared with two-screw fixation. However, others have demonstrated screws to have better torsional resistance to sagittal fibular translation.[115,116] Several systematic reviews have shown that SB fixation results in higher American Orthopedic Foot and Ankle Society (AOFAS) ankle-hindfoot scores and either similar or higher visual analog scale scores and Olerud-Molander Ankle Scores as compared with screw fixaton.[117–122] Additional benefits reported are lower malreduction rates, greater postoperative range of motion, earlier weightbearing, faster return to work and sport, and lower implant failure rates.[118–122] In one series, professional rugby players were able to return to sport after 2 months following SB fixation compared with 3 to 6 months following screw fixation.[123] Although Gan and colleagues[117] reported no difference in reoperation rates in their systematic review, others have reported lower failure and removal rates with SB fixation when excluding routine screw removal.[118–120]

The number and orientation of SB fixation are important surgical considerations. Frequently used constructs include one or two SBs placed axially in parallel or divergently.[115,124,125] Divergent fixation of double SBs may produce less diastasis, whereas parallel fixation better controlled fibular rotation in one cadaveric study.[125] Although biomechanical studies have demonstrated that multiple SB constructs provide stability comparable with single screw fixation,[115,124,125] there are conflicting reports regarding whether single SB constructs can sufficiently control sagittal fibular translation during rotation.[115,125–128] Although screw and SB fixation may overcompress the syndesmosis, a higher propensity to do so has been demonstrated with two SB fixation as compared with a single screw or SB.[124,129] Overcompression may not restrict ankle range of motion, but may alter kinematics or cause subtle talar subluxation.[130–132]

Although multiple biomechanical studies demonstrate comparable strength and stability between SBs and screws, to our knowledge no previous investigation has used a model where the fibula is length-unstable. SBs may be inadequate for certain injury patterns that require enhanced stability especially in the setting of axially unstable fractures (see **Fig. 7**B).[115,116] If fibular axial length is not restored by internal fixation, SB devices may be inadequate to prevent fibular shortening resulting in talar tilt and lateral talar displacement.[133] Furthermore, SB fixation is not without complications; several studies have reported medial neurovascular structure entrapment, osteolysis, and wound problems.[133–140]

Although the literature supports the use of SB fixation, implant cost (eg, list price) is significantly greater than typical metal screws. However, cost examined as total cost per episode of care better reflects the actual cost burden on the health care system. Several recent investigations have demonstrated relative cost effectiveness of SB devices depending on number of implants used, rates of comparative screw removal surgery, and associated operative costs.[4,122,123,141] Because surgical removal represents a cost and time burden on patients, SB fixation may be preferable for athletes.

SYNDESMOTIC LIGAMENT AUGMENTATION

There has been increased interest in adjunctive augmentation strategies. Although older investigations have examined the use of autograft or allograft tendon, newer techniques are being developed using nonabsorbable suture-tape materials.[142]

Syndesmotic Reconstruction Using Autograft/Allograft Tendon

The use of tendon graft to reconstruct the syndesmosis was first described by Castaing and colleagues[143] in 1961, using peroneus brevis tendon to reconstruct the AITFL and PITFL.[144–146] Various techniques have been described, but the general principle involves the creation of bone tunnels and passage of tendon graft to recreate various components of the syndesmotic ligamentous complex.

Isolated AITFL reconstruction has been described using various autograft and allograft sources.[144,147,148] Nelson[147] harvested a 6- to 8-cm graft of extensor digitorum longus tendon of the ipsilateral fourth toe and secured the graft to the ligamentous footprints using screws and washers. Yasui and colleagues[148] treated six patients with chronic instability using autograft gracilis tendon to reconstruct the AITFL after confirming integrity of the PITFL. After arthroscopic debridement, stabilization was achieved using a 3.5-mm screw.[148] Next, a 140-mm gracilis tendon was harvested from the ipsilateral knee and folded over itself twice.[148] Bone tunnels were created at the tibial and fibular AITFL foot prints and the graft was secured with a 5-mm interference screw.[148] At final follow-up, median AOFAS and visual analog scale scores improved from 53 to 95 and from 9.5 to 4, respectively.[148] Vilá-Rico and colleagues[144] describe a technique of using either gracilis or extensor hallucis longus allograft to reconstruct the syndesmosis through standard ankle arthroscopy portals without open reduction. After SB placement for stabilization,[144] tibial and fibular bone tunnels were created percutaneously. The prepared graft was then inserted through the anterolateral portal, passed through the tibial tunnel, and affixed using a tenodesis screw.[144] A suture was then used to pass the graft through the fibular bone tunnel, appropriately tensioned and affixed.[144]

Anterior Inferior Tibiofibular Ligament, Posterior Inferior Tibiofibular Ligament, and Interosseous Ligament Reconstruction

Several authors have described combined AITFL and PITFL reconstruction. Zamzani and Zamzam[149] reported on 11 patients treated for chronic instability using 10 cm of semitendinosus autograft from the ipsilateral knee. After initial arthroscopy, open reconstruction of the AITFL and PITFL was performed. At final assessment, 10 patients had complete resolution of pain and were able to return to their preinjury level of activity.[149] Che and colleagues[150] conducted a cadaveric study using a 12 to 15 cm length of peroneus brevis tendon. Their technique involved a total of four bone tunnels and passage of graft through the tunnels to form a single-bundle PITFL reconstruction and a double-bundle AITFL reconstruction.[150] When an ER force was applied, they found no significant difference in distal fibular displacement between the intact and reconstructed syndesmosis and between the reconstructed syndesmosis and tricortical screw fixation.[150] When a dorsiflexion force was applied, there was no significant difference in proximal fibular displacement between the intact and reconstructed models, although a difference was found between the reconstructed and screw-fixated model with screw fixation reducing proximal fibula displacement to 40% of the intact model.[150] These findings suggest that syndesmotic reconstruction may better approximate normal kinematics compared with screw fixation.[150]

Isolated reconstruction of the IOL has been described by Moravek and Kadakia[151] using semitendinosus allograft supplemented with SB fixation. Morris and colleagues[152] reviewed eight patients treated for chronic instability using screw fixation and semitendinosus autograft to reconstruct the AITFL and IOL. Following screw removal, patients were allowed to return to low-impact sporting activity with full return at 28 weeks postoperatively.[152] Seven patients were able to return to sports, although only four were able to return to their previous level.[152]

Colcuc and colleagues[145] conducted a retrospective review of 10 patients with grade III chronic isolated syndesmotic instability. Following syndesmotic fixation using a screw and SB construct, plantaris longus autograft was used to reconstruct the AITFL and IOL.[145] Weight bearing was allowed after screw removal at 8 weeks postoperatively.[145] Mean AOFAS scores increased from 53 ± 13 preoperatively to 86 ± 5 postoperatively and mean Weber scores increased from 12 ± 3 (poor) to 2 (good).

Some authors have reported results from complete syndesmotic reconstruction. Grass and colleagues[146] reviewed 16 patients treated using a modified version of Castaing's technique using splint peroneus longus tendon autograft (**Fig. 8**).[143] The syndesmotic screw was removed at 8 weeks postoperatively. At mean follow-up of 16.4 months, all patients demonstrated stability and 15 were near pain-free.[146] Despite promising results, the complexity of this technique has limited its adoption.[151,152]

Lui[153] more recently described a minimally invasive technique involving arthroscopic guidance and peroneus longus tendon autograft. The syndesmosis is similarly stabilized using a screw that is removed 8 weeks postoperatively.[153] The bone tunnels are created through the arthroscopic portals, and although the tibial tunnel is similar, the first fibular tunnel is made through the lateral malleolus to connect the fibular attachments of the AITFL and PITFL (**Fig. 9**). Reporting of outcomes is needed before widespread adoption.

Syndesmotic Ligament Reconstruction Using Nonabsorbable Suture-Tape

Increasingly, nonabsorbable knotless suture-tape has been used. Although extensive literature exists describing its use for lateral ligament augmentation, several reports have investigated its use for syndesmotic reconstruction.[154–171] The application of

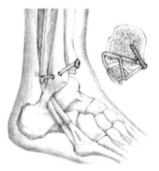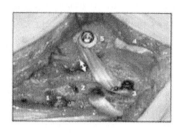

Fig. 8. Technique described by Grass and colleagues.[146] Three bone tunnels were drilled: one in the fibula at the level of the posterior tubercle and directed medially, cranially, and dorsally toward the posterior tibial tubercle; the second in the distal tibia originating from the posterior tubercle and directed anterolaterally toward the anterior tubercle; and the third in the fibula proximal to the other fibular tunnel and drilled from the lateral aspect of the fibula to meet the distal tibial tunnel. The free end of the detached proximal part of the peroneus longus tendon was then weaved through the tunnels and secured with a screw to reconstruct the syndesmosis as shown. (*From* Grass R, Rammelt S, Biewener A, Zwipp H. Peroneus longus ligamentoplasty for chronic instability of the distal tibiofibular syndesmosis. Foot Ankle Int. 2003; with permission.)

suture-tape for the treatment of syndesmotic injury was first reported by Mackay and colleagues[154] in 2015 followed by a more detailed description by Regauer and colleagues in 2017.[159] The concept is based on the use of suture-tape and knotless bone anchors to augment ligament healing (**Fig. 5E**).[159,172] The use of nonabsorbable knotless suture-tape has been described as a standalone treatment of augmentation of the AITFL or as a supplemental technique with SB fixation.[159,161,162] The standalone technique described by Regauer and colleagues[159] is used for augmentation of the AITFL and PITFL, although it is easily adapted for single ligament reconstruction. Harris and colleagues[160] reported treating 11 athletes, although it is unclear whether one

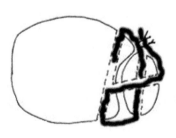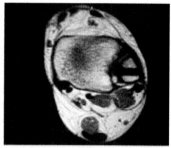

Fig. 9. Minimally invasive technique described by Lui.[153] The first fibular tunnel is made through the lateral malleolus to connect the fibular attachments of the AITFL and PITFL. The second fibular tunnel is made directly lateral just above the level of the tibial tunnel and directed posteromedially to join the tibial tunnel. One end of the graft is passed from the posterior end of the tibial tunnel and pulled through the interosseous fibular tunnel. The other end of the graft is then passed from the posterior fibula to the anterior fibula and then placed into distal tibial tunnel. The stay stitch of the posterolateral incision is then brought to the anterolateral incision and sutured to the graft with the graft in tension.[153] (*From* Lui TH. Tri-ligamentous reconstruction of the distal tibiofibular syndesmosis: A minimally invasive approach. J Foot Ankle Surg. 2010;49(5):495-500; with permission.)

or both the AITFL and PITFL were augmented. All patients had a final AOFAS score of 100, although preoperative scores were not reported.[160] Nine patients were able to return to play within 12 weeks and had full dorsiflexion as demonstrated by the knee-to-wall test.[160] Other case reports have been published using nonabsorbable knotless suture-tape in conjunction with SB fixation.[159,162,163]

Shoji and colleagues[161] performed a biomechanical study comparing the stability of SB fixation, SB fixation augmented with suture-tape, suture-tape alone, or screw fixation alone. When an anterior traction force was applied to represent ankle dorsiflexion, SB fixation alone resulted in a significant increase in tibiofibular diastasis and fibular rotation angle compared with the intact syndesmosis.[161] However, SB fixation augmented with suture-tape, suture-tape alone, and screw fixation did not demonstrate significant changes in tibiofibular diastasis or fibular rotation angle.[161] Ultimately, screw fixation was more rigid compared with the intact model, but ST augmentation of SB fixation achieved dynamic stability similar to intact models.[161] Augmentation with nonabsorbable knotless suture-tape is a promising technique for either acute or chronic syndesmotic fixation.

Arthrodesis

Although the current literature is limited, arthrodesis may be a suitable salvage procedure in cases of chronic instability accompanied by arthrosis (**Fig. 6**).[173] Pena and Coetzee recommend arthrodesis for patients with chronic symptoms, severe incongruency, or recurrent diastasis after screw removal.[173] Typically an anterolateral approach is used,[173–176] although arthroscopy may be used to aid debridement.[177,178] Basic surgical principles for joint arthrodesis are followed, including debridement, decortication, bone grafting, and rigid internal fixation. Patients are casted and should remain nonweightbearing until bony fusion occurs typically within 6 to 10 weeks.[173–176] Patients are then progressed full weightbearing.[173–176] In a cohort of 10 patients, Olson and colleagues[174] reported mean AOFAS scores increased from 37 ± 15 preoperatively to 87 ± 11 postoperatively at average follow-up of 41 months. There was no change in ankle range of motion, although this may have been confounded by seven patients undergoing concomitant Achilles lengthening. All patients reported satisfaction and would undergo the procedure again.[174]

SUMMARY

Acute and chronic syndesmotic injuries can significantly impact athletic function and activities of daily living. Patient history, examination, and the judicious use of imaging modalities aid diagnosis. Surgical management should be used when frank diastasis, instability, and/or chronic pain and disability ensues.

DISCLOSURE

J.Y. Kwon: Paragon 28: IP royalties; paid consultant.

REFERENCES

1. Shibuya N, Davis ML, Jupiter DC. Epidemiology of foot and ankle fractures in the United States: an analysis of the National Trauma Data Bank (2007 to 2011). J Foot Ankle Surg 2014;53(5):606–8.

2. Jennison T, Brinsden M. Fracture admission trends in England over a ten-year period. Ann R Coll Surg Engl 2019;101(3):208–14.

3. Dattani R, Patnaik S, Kantak A, et al. Injuries to the tibiofibular syndesmosis. J Bone Joint Surg Br 2008;90(4):405–10.

4. Ramsey DC, Friess DM. Cost-effectiveness analysis of syndesmotic screw versus suture button fixation in tibiofibular syndesmotic injuries. J Orthop Trauma 2018;32(6):e198–203.

5. Hootman JM, Dick R, Agel J. Epidemiology of collegiate injuries for 15 sports: summary and recommendations for injury prevention initiatives. J Athl Train 2007;42(2):311–9.

6. Fong DTP, Hong Y, Chan LK, et al. A systematic review on ankle injury and ankle sprain in sports. Sports Med 2007;37(1):73–94.

7. Williams BT, Ahrberg AB, Goldsmith MT, et al. Ankle syndesmosis: a qualitative and quantitative anatomic analysis. Am J Sports Med 2015;43(1):88–97.

8. Vosseller JT, Karl JW, Greisberg JK. Incidence of syndesmotic injury. Orthopedics 2014;37(3):226–30.

9. Hunt KJ, Phisitkul P, Pirolo J, et al. High ankle sprains and syndesmotic injuries in athletes. J Am Acad Orthop Surg 2015;23(11):661–73.

10. Gerber JP, Williams GN, Scoville CR, et al. Persistent disability associated with ankle sprains: a prospective examination of an athletic population. Foot Ankle Int 1998;19(10):653–60.

11. White T, Bugler K. Ankle fractures. In: Tornetta IIIP, Ricci WM, Ostrum RF, et al, editors. Rockwood and Green's fractures in adults. 9th edition. Philadelphia: Wolters Kluwer; 2020. p. 2822–76.

12. Weening B, Bhandari M. Predictors of functional outcome following transsyndesmotic screw fixation of ankle fractures. J Orthop Trauma 2005;19(2):102–8.

13. Kennedy JG, Soffe KE, Vedova PD, et al. Evaluation of the syndesmotic screw in low Weber C ankle fractures. J Orthop Trauma 2000. https://doi.org/10.1097/00005131-200006000-00010.

14. Sagi HC, Shah AR, Sanders RW. The functional consequence of syndesmotic joint malreduction at a minimum 2-year follow-up. J Orthop Trauma 2012. https://doi.org/10.1097/BOT.0b013e31822a526a.

15. Ray R, Koohnejad N, Clement ND, et al. Ankle fractures with syndesmotic stabilisation are associated with a high rate of secondary osteoarthritis. Foot Ankle Surg 2019;25(2):180–5.

16. Hermans JJ, Beumer A, de Jong TAW, et al. Anatomy of the distal tibiofibular syndesmosis in adults: a pictorial essay with a multimodality approach. J Anat 2010;217(6):633–45.

17. Boszczyk A, Kwapisz S, Krümmel M, et al. Correlation of incisura anatomy with syndesmotic malreduction. Foot Ankle Int 2018;39(3):369–75. Available at: http://limo.libis.be/resolver?&sid=EMBASE&issn=19447876&id=doi:10.1177%2F1071100717744332&atitle=Correlation+of+Incisura+Anatomy+With+Syndesmotic+Malreduction&stitle=Foot+Ankle+Int.&title=Foot+and+Ankle+International&volume=39&issue=3&spage=369&epage=375&aulast=Boszczyk&aufirst=Andrzej&auinit=A.&aufull=Boszczyk+A.&coden=FAINE&isbn=&pages=369-375&date=2018&auinit1=A&auinitm=.

18. Panchbhavi VK, Gurbani BN, Mason CB, et al. Radiographic assessment of fibular length variance: the case for "fibula minus". J Foot Ankle Surg 2018;57(1):91–4.

19. Bartoníček J. Anatomy of the tibiofibular syndesmosis and its clinical relevance. Surg Radiol Anat 2003;25(5–6):379–86.

20. Ogilvie-Harris DJ, Reed SC, Hedman TP. Disruption of the ankle syndesmosis: biomechanical study of the ligamentous restraints. Arthroscopy 1994;10(5): 558–60.
21. Haraguchi N, Haruyama H, Toga H, et al. Pathoanatomy of posterior malleolar fractures of the ankle. J Bone Joint Surg Am 2006;88(5):1085–92.
22. Fitzpatrick E, Goetz JE, Sittapairoj T, et al. Effect of posterior malleolus fracture on syndesmotic reduction: a cadaveric study. J Bone Joint Surg Am 2018; 100(3):243–8.
23. Miller AN, Carroll EA, Parker RJ, et al. Posterior malleolar stabilization of syndesmotic injuries is equivalent to screw fixation. Clin Orthop Relat Res 2010;468(4): 1129–35.
24. Kang C, Hwang D-S, Lee J-K, et al. Screw fixation of the posterior malleolus fragment in ankle fracture. Foot Ankle Int 2019. https://doi.org/10.1177/1071100719865895. 1071100719865895.
25. McKeon KE, Wright RW, Johnson JE, et al. Vascular anatomy of the tibiofibular syndesmosis. J Bone Joint Surg Am 2012;94:931–8.
26. Jeong MS, Choi YS, Kim YJ, et al. Deltoid ligament in acute ankle injury: MR imaging analysis. Skeletal Radiol 2014;43(5):655–63.
27. Massri-Pugin J, Lubberts B, Vopat BG, et al. Role of the deltoid ligament in syndesmotic instability. Foot Ankle Int 2018;39(5):598–603.
28. Massri-Pugin J, Lubberts B, Vopat BG, et al. Effect of sequential sectioning of ligaments on syndesmotic instability in the coronal plane evaluated arthroscopically. Foot Ankle Int 2017;38(12):1387–93.
29. Goetz JE, Vasseenon T, Tochigi Y, et al. 3D talar kinematics during external rotation stress testing in hindfoot varus and valgus using a model of syndesmotic and deep deltoid instability. Foot Ankle Int 2019;40(7):826–35.
30. Sman AD, Hiller CE, Refshauge KM. Diagnostic accuracy of clinical tests for diagnosis of ankle syndesmosis injury: a systematic review. Br J Sports Med 2013;47(10):620–8.
31. Ebraheim NA, Elgafy H, Padanilam T. Syndesmotic disruption in low fibular fractures associated with deltoid ligament injury. Clin Orthop Relat Res 2003. https://doi.org/10.1097/01.blo.0000052935.71325.30.
32. Mauntel TC, Wikstrom EA, Roos KG, et al. The epidemiology of high ankle sprains in National Collegiate Athletic Association sports. Am J Sports Med 2017;45(9):2156–63.
33. Williams GN, Jones MH, Amendola A. Syndesmotic ankle sprains in athletes. Am J Sports Med 2007;35(7):1197–207.
34. Hunt KJ. Syndesmosis injuries. Curr Rev Musculoskelet Med 2013;6(4):304–12.
35. van Dijk CN, Longo UG, Loppini M, et al. Classification and diagnosis of acute isolated syndesmotic injuries: ESSKA-AFAS consensus and guidelines. Knee Surg Sports Traumatol Arthrosc 2016;24(4):1200–16.
36. Switaj PJ, Mendoza M, Kadakia AR. Acute and chronic injuries to the syndesmosis. Clin Sports Med 2015;34(4):643–77.
37. van den Bekerom MPJ, de Leeuw PAJ, van Dijk CN. Delayed operative treatment of syndesmotic instability. Current concepts review. Injury 2009;40(11): 1137–42.
38. Espinosa N, Smerek JP, Myerson MS. Acute and chronic syndesmosis injuries: pathomechanisms, diagnosis and management. Foot Ankle Clin 2006;11(3): 639–57.

39. Scranton PE, McDermott JE, Rogers JV. The relationship between chronic ankle instability and variations in mortise anatomy and impingement spurs. Foot Ankle Int 2000;21(8):657–64.

40. Knapik DM, Trem A, Sheehan J, et al. Conservative management for stable high ankle injuries in professional football players. Sports Health 2018;10(1):80–4.

41. Calder JD, Bamford R, Petrie A, et al. Stable versus unstable grade II high ankle sprains: a prospective study predicting the need for surgical stabilization and time to return to sports. Arthroscopy 2016;32(4):634–42.

42. D'Hooghe P, Grassi A, Alkhelaifi K, et al. Return to play after surgery for isolated unstable syndesmotic ankle injuries (West Point grade IIB and III) in 110 male professional football players: a retrospective cohort study. Br J Sports Med 2019. https://doi.org/10.1136/bjsports-2018-100298.

43. Oae K, Takao M, Naito K, et al. Injury of the tibiofibular syndesmosis: value of MR imaging for diagnosis. Radiology 2003;227(1):155–61.

44. Hagemeijer NC, Chang SH, Abdelaziz ME, et al. Range of normal and abnormal syndesmotic measurements using weightbearing CT. Foot Ankle Int 2019. https://doi.org/10.1177/1071100719866831. 1071100719866831.

45. Harper MC, Keller TS. A radiographic evaluation of the tibiofibular syndesmosis. Foot Ankle 1989;10(3):156–60.

46. Shah AS, Kadakia AR, Tan GJ, et al. Radiographic evaluation of the normal distal tibiofibular syndesmosis. Foot Ankle Int 2012;33(10):870–6.

47. Marmor M, Hansen E, Han HK, et al. Limitations of standard fluoroscopy in detecting rotational malreduction of the syndesmosis in an ankle fracture model. Foot Ankle Int 2011;32(6):616–22.

48. Matuszewski PE, Dombroski D, Lawrence JTR, et al. Prospective intraoperative syndesmotic evaluation during ankle fracture fixation: stress external rotation versus lateral fibular stress. J Orthop Trauma 2015;29(4):e157–60.

49. Jiang KN, Schulz BM, Tsui YL, et al. Comparison of radiographic stress tests for syndesmotic instability of supination-external rotation ankle fractures: a cadaveric study. J Orthop Trauma 2014;28(6):e123–7.

50. Saldua NS, Harris JF, LeClere LE, et al. Plantar flexion influences radiographic measurements of the ankle mortise. J Bone Joint Surg Am 2010;92(4):911–5.

51. Park SS, Kubiak EN, Egol KA, et al. Stress radiographs after ankle fracture: the effect of ankle position and deltoid ligament status on medial clear space measurements. J Orthop Trauma 2006;20(1):11–8. Available at: http://www.ncbi.nlm.nih.gov/pubmed/16424804.

52. Nault M-L, Hébert-Davies J, Laflamme G-Y, et al. CT scan assessment of the syndesmosis: a new reproducible method. J Orthop Trauma 2013;27(11):638–41. Available at: www.jorthotrauma.com.

53. Ebraheim NA, Lu J, Yang H, et al. Radiographic and CT evaluation of tibiofibular syndesmotic diastasis: a cadaver study. Foot Ankle Int 1997;18(11):693–8.

54. Malhotra G, Cameron J, Toolan BC. Diagnosing chronic diastasis of the syndesmosis: a novel measurement using computed tomography. Foot Ankle Int 2014;35(5):483–8.

55. Patel S, Malhotra K, Cullen NP, et al. Defining reference values for the normal tibiofibular syndesmosis in adults using weight-bearing CT. Bone Joint J 2019;101-B(3):348–52.

56. Han SH, Lee JW, Kim S, et al. Chronic tibiofibular syndesmosis injury: the diagnostic efficiency of magnetic resonance imaging and comparative analysis of operative treatment. Foot Ankle Int 2007;28(3):336–42.

57. Ryan LP, Hills MC, Chang J, et al. The lambda sign: a new radiographic indicator of latent syndesmosis instability. Foot Ankle Int 2014;35(9):903–8.
58. Lui TH, Ip K, Chow HT. Comparison of radiologic and arthroscopic diagnoses of distal tibiofibular syndesmosis disruption in acute ankle fracture. Arthroscopy 2005;21(11):1370.
59. Guyton GP, DeFontes K, Barr CR, et al. Arthroscopic correlates of subtle syndesmotic injury. Foot Ankle Int 2017;38(5):502–6.
60. Lubberts B, Massri-Pugin J, Guss D, et al. Arthroscopic assessment of syndesmotic instability in the sagittal plane in a cadaveric model. Foot Ankle Int 2019. https://doi.org/10.1177/1071100719879673. 1071100719879673.
61. Miller AN, Carroll EA, Parker RJ, et al. Direct visualization for syndesmotic stabilization of ankle fractures. Foot Ankle Int 2009;30(5):419–26.
62. Gardner MJ, Demetrakopoulos D, Briggs SM, et al. Malreduction of the tibiofibular syndesmosis in ankle fractures. Foot Ankle Int 2006;27(10):788–92.
63. LaMothe J, Baxter JR, Gilbert S, et al. Effect of complete syndesmotic disruption and deltoid injuries and different reduction methods on ankle joint contact mechanics. Foot Ankle Int 2017;38(6):694–700.
64. Gardner MJ, Demetrakopoulos D, Briggs SM, et al. Malreduction of the tibiofibular syndesmosis in ankle fractures. Foot Ankle Int;27(10):788 to 792.
65. Tornetta P, Yakavonis M, Veltre D, et al. Reducing the syndesmosis under direct vision: where should I look? J Orthop Trauma 2019;33(9):450–4.
66. Miller AN, Barei DP, Iaquinto JM, et al. Iatrogenic syndesmosis malreduction via clamp and screw placement. J Orthop Trauma 2013;27(2):100–6. Available at: www.jorthotrauma.com.
67. Cosgrove CT, Putnam SM, Cherney SM, et al. Medial clamp tine positioning affects ankle syndesmosis malreduction. J Orthop Trauma 2017;31:440–6. Lippincott Williams and Wilkins.
68. Park YH, Ahn JH, Choi GW, et al. Comparison of clamp reduction and manual reduction of syndesmosis in rotational ankle fractures: a prospective randomized trial. J Foot Ankle Surg 2018;57(1):19–22.
69. Franke J, von Recum J, Suda AJ, et al. Intraoperative three-dimensional imaging in the treatment of acute unstable syndesmotic injuries. J Bone Joint Surg Am 2012;94(15):1386–90.
70. Hansen M, Le L, Wertheimer S, et al. Syndesmosis fixation: analysis of shear stress via axial load on 3.5-mm and 4.5-mm quadricortical syndesmotic screws. J Foot Ankle Surg 2006;45(2):65–9.
71. Thompson MC, Gesink DS. Biomechenical comparison of syndesmosis fixation with 3.5- and 4.5-millimeter stainless steel screws. Foot Ankle Int 2000;21(9): 736–41.
72. Markolf KL, Jackson SR, McAllister DR. Syndesmosis fixation using dual 3.5 mm and 4.5 mm screws with tricortical and quadricortical purchase: a biomechanical study. Foot Ankle Int 2013;34(5):734–9.
73. Stuart K, Panchbhavi VK. The fate of syndesmotic screws. Foot Ankle Int 2011; 32(5):S519–25.
74. Lee SY, Moon SY, Park MS, et al. Syndesmosis fixation in unstable ankle fractures using a partially threaded 5.0-mm cannulated screw. J Foot Ankle Surg 2018;57(4):721–5.
75. Stenquist D, Velasco BT, Cronin PK, et al. Syndesmotic fixation utilizing a novel screw: a retrospective case series reporting early clinical and radiographic outcomes. Foot Ankle Spec 2019. https://doi.org/10.1177/1938640019866322. 193864001986632.

76. Moore JA, Shank JR, Morgan SJ, et al. Syndesmosis fixation: a comparison of three and four cortices of screw fixation without hardware removal. Foot Ankle Int 2006;27(8):567–72.

77. Serhan M, Verim O, Altinel L, et al. Three-dimensional finite element analysis used to compare six different methods of syndesmosis fixation with 3.5- or 4.5-mm titanium screws: a biomechanical study. J Am Podiatr Med Assoc 2013;103(3):174–80.

78. Høiness P, Strømsøe K. Tricortical versus quadricortical syndesmosis fixation in ankle fractures: a prospective, randomized study comparing two methods of syndesmosis fixation. J Orthop Trauma 2004;18(6):331–7.

79. Li H, Chen Y, Qiang M, et al. Computational biomechanical analysis of postoperative inferior tibiofibular syndesmosis: a modified modeling method. Comput Methods Biomech Biomed Engin 2018;21(5):427–35.

80. Peek AC, Fitzgerald CE, Charalambides C. Syndesmosis screws: how many, what diameter, where and should they be removed? A literature review. Injury 2014;45(8):1262–7.

81. Michelson JD, Wright M, Blankstein M. Syndesmotic ankle fractures. J Orthop Trauma 2018;32(1):10–4.

82. Hahn DM, Chong K. Malleoli. In: Buckley RE, Moran CG, Apivatthakakul T, editors. AO principles of fracture management. 3rd edition. Davos Platz (Switzerland): AO Publishing; 2017. p. 933–60.

83. Mendelsohn ES, Hoshino CM, Harris TG, et al. CT characterizing the anatomy of uninjured ankle syndesmosis. Orthopedics 2014;37(2):157–61.

84. Cosgrove CT, Spraggs-Hughes AG, Putnam SM, et al. A novel indirect reduction technique in ankle syndesmotic injuries: a cadaveric study. J Orthop Trauma 2018;32(7):361–7.

85. Kukreti S, Faraj A, Miles JNV. Does position of syndesmotic screw affect functional and radiological outcome in ankle fractures? Injury 2005;36(9):1121–4.

86. McBryde A, Chiasson B, Wilhelm A, et al. Syndesmotic screw placement: a biomechanical analysis. Foot Ankle Int 1997;18(5):262–6.

87. Miller RS. Comparison of tricortical screw fixation versus a modified suture construct for fixation of ankle syndesmosis injury: a biomechanical study. J Orthop Trauma 1998. https://doi.org/10.1097/00005131-199901000-00009.

88. Tile M. Fractures of the ankle. In: Schatzker J, Tile M, editors. The rationale of operative fracture care. 3rd Edition. Berlin: Springer; 2005. p. 551–90.

89. Bava E, Charlton T, Thordarson D. Ankle fracture syndesmosis fixation and management: the current practice of orthopedic surgeons. Am J Orthop (Belle Mead NJ) 2010;39(5):242–6. http://www.ncbi.nlm.nih.gov/pubmed/20567742.

90. Schepers T, Van Zuuren WJ, Van Den Bekerom MPJ, et al. The management of acute distal tibio-fibular syndesmotic injuries: results of a nationwide survey. Injury 2012;43(10):1718–23.

91. Huber T, Schmoelz W, Bölderl A. Motion of the fibula relative to the tibia and its alterations with syndesmosis screws: a cadaver study. Foot Ankle Surg 2012; 18(3):203–9.

92. Manjoo A, Sanders DW, Tieszer C, et al. Functional and radiographic results of patients with syndesmotic screw fixation: implications for screw removal. J Orthop Trauma 2010;24(1):2–6.

93. Briceno J, Wusu T, Kaiser P, et al. Effect of syndesmotic implant removal on dorsiflexion. Foot Ankle Int 2019. https://doi.org/10.1177/1071100718818572.

94. Dingemans SA, Rammelt S, White TO, et al. Should syndesmotic screws be removed after surgical fixation of unstable ankle fractures? A systematic review. Bone Joint J 2016;98-B(11):1497–504.

95. Walley KC, Hofmann KJ, Velasco BT, et al. Removal of hardware after syndesmotic screw fixation: a systematic literature review. Foot Ankle Spec 2017; 10(3):252–7.

96. Thordarson DB, Samuelson M, Shepherd LE, et al. Bioabsorbable versus stainless steel screw fixation of the syndesmosis in pronation-lateral rotation ankle fractures: a prospective randomized trial. Foot Ankle Int 2001;22(4):335–8.

97. Hovis WD, Kaiser BW, Watson JT, et al. Treatment of syndesmotic disruptions of the ankle with bioabsorbable screw fixation. J Bone Joint Surg Am 2002;84(1): 26–31.

98. Sinisaari IP, Lüthje PMJ, Mikkonen RHM. Ruptured tibio-fibular syndesmosis: comparison study of metallic to bioabsorbable fixation. Foot Ankle Int 2002; 23(8):744–8.

99. Cox S, Mukherjee DP, Ogden AL, et al. Distal tibiofibular syndesmosis fixation: a cadaveric, simulated fracture stabilization study comparing bioabsorbable and metallic single screw fixation. J Foot Ankle Surg 2005;44(2):144–51.

100. Kaukonen JP, Lamberg T, Korkala O, et al. Fixation of syndesmotic ruptures in 38 patients with a malleolar fracture: a randomized study comparing a metallic and a bioabsorbable screw. J Orthop Trauma 2005;19(6):392–5.

101. Ahmad J, Raikin SM, Pour AE, et al. Bioabsorbable screw fixation of the syndesmosis in unstable ankle injuries. Foot Ankle Int 2009;30(2):99–105.

102. Sun H, Luo CF, Zhong B, et al. A prospective, randomised trial comparing the use of absorbable and metallic screws in the fixation of distal tibiofibular syndesmosis injuries: mid-term follow-up. Bone Joint J 2014;96 B(4):548–54.

103. Blasier RD, Bucholz R, Cole W, et al. Bioresorbable implants: applications in orthopaedic surgery. Instr Course Lect 1997;46:531–46.

104. Hovis WD, Watson JT, Bucholz RW. Biochemical and biomechanical properties of bioabsorbable implants used in fracture fixation. Tech Orthop 1998. https://doi.org/10.1097/00013611-199806000-00005.

105. Xie Y, Cai L, Deng Z, et al. Absorbable screws versus metallic screws for distal tibiofibular syndesmosis injuries: a meta-analysis. J Foot Ankle Surg 2015;54(4): 663–70.

106. van der Eng DM, Schep NWL, Schepers T. Bioabsorbable versus metallic screw fixation for tibiofibular syndesmotic ruptures: a meta-analysis. J Foot Ankle Surg 2015;54(4):657–62.

107. Böstman O, Pihlajamäki H. Clinical biocompatibility of biodegradable orthopaedic implants for internal fixation: a review. Biomaterials 2000;21(24):2615–21.

108. Thordarson DB, Hedman TP, Gross D, et al. Biomechanical evaluation of polylactide absorbable screws used for syndesmosis injury repair. Foot Ankle Int 1997;18(10):622–7.

109. Liu G, Chen L, Gong M, et al. Clinical evidence for treatment of distal tibiofibular syndesmosis injury: a systematic review of clinical studies. J Foot Ankle Surg 2019;1–6. https://doi.org/10.1053/j.jfas.2019.01.015.

110. Petrisor BA, Poolman R, Koval K, et al. Management of displaced ankle fractures. J Orthop Trauma 2006. https://doi.org/10.1097/00005131-200608000-00012.

111. Bostman OM. Intense granulomatous inflammatory lesions associated with absorbable internal fixation devices made of polyglycolide in ankle fractures.

Clin Orthop Relat Res 1992. https://doi.org/10.1097/00003086-199205000-00031.

112. Böstman O, Partio E, Hirvensalo E, et al. Foreign-body reactions to polyglycolide screws: observations in 24/216 malleolar fracture cases. Acta Orthop 1992. https://doi.org/10.3109/17453679209154817.

113. Hovis WD, Bucholz RW. Polyglycolide bioabsorbable screws in the treatment of ankle fractures. Foot Ankle Int 1997. https://doi.org/10.1177/107110079701800303.

114. Pang EQ, Bedigrew K, Palanca A, et al. Ankle joint contact loads and displacement in syndesmosis injuries repaired with Tightropes compared to screw fixation in a static model. Injury 2019;1–7. https://doi.org/10.1016/j.injury.2019.09.012.

115. Clanton TO, Whitlow SR, Williams BT, et al. Biomechanical comparison of 3 current ankle syndesmosis repair techniques. Foot Ankle Int 2017;38(2):200–7.

116. Ebramzadeh E, Knutsen AR, Sangiorgio SN, et al. Biomechanical comparison of syndesmotic injury fixation methods using a cadaveric model. Foot Ankle Int 2013;34(12):1710–7.

117. Gan K, Xu D, Hu K, et al. Dynamic fixation is superior in terms of clinical outcomes to static fixation in managing distal tibiofibular syndesmosis injury. Knee Surg Sports Traumatol Arthrosc 2019. https://doi.org/10.1007/s00167-019-05659-0.

118. McKenzie AC, Hesselholt KE, Larsen MS, et al. A systematic review and meta-analysis on treatment of ankle fractures with syndesmotic rupture: suture-button fixation versus cortical screw fixation. J Foot Ankle Surg 2019;58(5):946–53.

119. Grassi A, Samuelsson K, D'Hooghe P, et al. Dynamic stabilization of syndesmosis injuries reduces complications and reoperations as compared with screw fixation: a meta-analysis of randomized controlled trials. Am J Sports Med 2019;1–14. https://doi.org/10.1177/0363546519849909.

120. Chen BH, Chen C, Yang ZT, et al. To compare the efficacy between fixation with tightrope and screw in the treatment of syndesmotic injuries: a meta-analysis. Foot Ankle Surg 2019;25(1):63–70.

121. Shimozono Y, Hurley ET, Myerson CL, et al. Suture button versus syndesmotic screw for syndesmosis injuries: a meta-analysis of randomized controlled trials. Am J Sports Med 2018. https://doi.org/10.1177/0363546518804804. 363546518804804.

122. Zhang P, Liang Y, He J, et al. A systematic review of suture-button versus syndesmotic screw in the treatment of distal tibiofibular syndesmosis injury. BMC Musculoskelet Disord 2017;18(1):1–12.

123. Latham AJ, Goodwin PC, Stirling B, et al. Ankle syndesmosis repair and rehabilitation in professional rugby league players: a case series report. BMJ Open Sport Exerc Med 2017;3(1):1–6.

124. Schon JM, Williams BT, Venderley MB, et al. A 3-D CT analysis of screw and suture-button fixation of the syndesmosis. Foot Ankle Int 2017;38(2):208–14.

125. Parker AS, Beason DP, Slowik JS, et al. Biomechanical comparison of 3 syndesmosis repair techniques with suture button implants. Orthop J Sport Med 2018; 6(10):1–6.

126. Lamothe JM, Baxter JR, Murphy C, et al. Three-dimensional analysis of fibular motion after fixation of syndesmotic injuries with a screw or suture-button construct. Foot Ankle Int 2016. https://doi.org/10.1177/1071100716666865.

127. Soin SP, Knight TA, Dinah AF, et al. Suture-button versus screw fixation in a syndesmosis rupture model: a biomechanical comparison. Foot Ankle Int 2009. https://doi.org/10.3113/FAI.2009.0346.

128. Klitzman RG, Zhao H, Zhang LQ, et al. Suture-button versus screw fixation of the syndesmosis: a biomechanical analysis. Foot Ankle Int 2010. https://doi.org/10.3113/FAI.2010.0069.

129. Schon JM, Mikula JD, Backus JD, et al. 3D model analysis of ankle flexion on anatomic reduction of a syndesmotic injury. Foot Ankle Int 2017;38(4):436–42.

130. Gonzalez T, Egan J, Ghorbanhoseini M, et al. Overtightening of the syndesmosis revisited and the effect of syndesmotic malreduction on ankle dorsiflexion. Injury 2017;48(6):1253–7.

131. Tornetta P, Spoo JE, Reynolds FA, et al. Overtightening of the ankle syndesmosis: is it really possible? J Bone Joint Surg Am 2001. https://doi.org/10.2106/00004623-200104000-00002.

132. Mahapatra P, Rudge B, Whittingham-Jones P. Is it possible to overcompress the syndesmosis? J Foot Ankle Surg 2018;57(5):1005–9.

133. Riedel MD, Miller CP, Kwon JY. Augmenting suture-button fixation for maisonneuve injuries with fibular shortening: technique tip. Foot Ankle Int 2017; 38(10):1146–51.

134. Pirozzi KM, Creech CL, Meyr AJ. Assessment of anatomic risk during syndesmotic stabilization with the suture button technique. J Foot Ankle Surg 2015; 54(5):917–9.

135. Lehtonen EJ, Pinto MC, Patel HA, et al. Syndesmotic fixation with suture button: neurovascular structures at risk: a cadaver study. Foot Ankle Spec 2019. https://doi.org/10.1177/1938640019826699.

136. Reb CW, Brandão RA, Watson BC, et al. Medial structure injury during suture button insertion using the center-center technique for syndesmotic stabilization. Foot Ankle Int 2018;39(8):984–9.

137. Willmott HJS, Singh B, David LA. Outcome and complications of treatment of ankle diastasis with tightrope fixation. Injury 2009. https://doi.org/10.1016/j.injury.2009.05.008.

138. DeGroot H, Al-Omari AA, El Ghazaly SA. Outcomes of suture button repair of the distal tibiofibular syndesmosis. Foot Ankle Int 2011. https://doi.org/10.3113/FAI.2011.0250.

139. Storey P, Gadd RJ, Blundell C, et al. Complications of suture button ankle syndesmosis stabilization with modifications of surgical technique. Foot Ankle Int 2012. https://doi.org/10.3113/FAI.2012.0717.

140. Naqvi GA, Shafqat A, Awan N. Tightrope fixation of ankle syndesmosis injuries: clinical outcome, complications and technique modification. Injury 2012. https://doi.org/10.1016/j.injury.2011.10.002.

141. Weber AC, Hull MG, Johnson AJ, et al. Cost analysis of ankle syndesmosis internal fixation. J Clin Orthop Trauma 2019;10(1):173–7.

142. Goetz JE, Davidson NP, Rudert MJ, et al. Biomechanical comparison of syndesmotic repair techniques during external rotation stress. Foot Ankle Int 2018; 39(11):1345–54.

143. Castaing J, Le Chevallier P, Meunier M. Entorse à répétition ou subluxation récidivante de la tibio-tarsienne. Une technique simple de ligamentoplastie externe. Rev Chir Orthop Reparatrice Appar Mot 1961.

144. Vilá-Rico J, Sánchez-Morata E, Vacas-Sánchez E, et al. Anatomical arthroscopic graft reconstruction of the anterior tibiofibular ligament for chronic disruption of the distal syndesmosis. Arthrosc Tech 2018;7(2):e165–9.

145. Colcuc C, Fischer S, Colcuc S, et al. Treatment strategies for partial chronic instability of the distal syndesmosis: an arthroscopic grading scale and operative staging concept. Arch Orthop Trauma Surg 2016;136(2):157–63.

146. Grass R, Rammelt S, Biewener A, et al. Peroneus longus ligamentoplasty for chronic instability of the distal tibiofibular syndesmosis. Foot Ankle Int 2003.

147. Nelson OA. Examination and repair of the AITFL in transmalleolar fractures. J Orthop Trauma 2006;20(9):637–43.

148. Yasui Y, Takao M, Miyamoto W, et al. Anatomical reconstruction of the anterior inferior tibiofibular ligament for chronic disruption of the distal tibiofibular syndesmosis. Knee Surgery. Sport Traumatol Arthrosc 2011;19(4):691–5.

149. Zamzami MM, Zamzam MM. Chronic isolated distal tibiofibular syndesmotic disruption: diagnosis and management. Foot Ankle Surg 2009;15(1):14–9.

150. Che J, Li C, Gao Z, et al. Novel anatomical reconstruction of distal tibiofibular ligaments restores syndesmotic biomechanics. Knee Surg Sports Traumatol Arthrosc 2017;25(6):1866–72.

151. Moravek JE, Kadakia AR. Surgical strategies: doubled allograft reconstruction for chronic syndesmotic injuries. Foot Ankle Int 2010;31(9):834–44.

152. Morris MWJ, Rice P, Schneider TE. Distal tibiofibular syndesmosis reconstruction using a free hamstring autograft. Foot Ankle Int 2009;30(6):506–11.

153. Lui TH. Tri-ligamentous reconstruction of the distal tibiofibular syndesmosis: a minimally invasive approach. J Foot Ankle Surg 2010;49(5):495–500.

154. Mackay GM, Blyth MJG, Anthony I, et al. A review of ligament augmentation with the InternalBrace™: the surgical principle is described for the lateral ankle ligament and ACL repair in particular, and a comprehensive review of other surgical applications and techniques is presented. Surg Technol Int 2015;26:239–55.

155. Cho BK, Park KJ, Kim SW, et al. Minimal invasive suture-tape augmentation for chronic ankle instability. Foot Ankle Int 2015. https://doi.org/10.1177/1071100715592217.

156. Cho BK, Hong SH, Jeon JH. Effect of lateral ligament augmentation using suture-tape on functional ankle instability. Foot Ankle Int 2019. https://doi.org/10.1177/1071100718818554.

157. Cho BK, Park JK, Choi SM, et al. A randomized comparison between lateral ligaments augmentation using suture-tape and modified Broström repair in young female patients with chronic ankle instability. Foot Ankle Surg 2019. https://doi.org/10.1016/j.fas.2017.09.008.

158. Ulku TK, Kocaoglu B, Tok O, et al. Arthroscopic suture-tape internal bracing is safe as arthroscopic modified Broström repair in the treatment of chronic ankle instability. Knee Surg Sports Traumatol Arthrosc 2019. https://doi.org/10.1007/s00167-019-05552-w.

159. Regauer M, Mackay G, Lange M, et al. Syndesmotic Internal Brace™ for anatomic distal tibiofibular ligament augmentation. World J Orthop 2017;8(4):301–9.

160. Harris N, Farndon M, Hannant G. Stabilisation of the ankle syndesmosis using the Internal Brace (Arthrex). In: British Orthopaedic Foot and Ankle Society Annual Meeting. Edinburgh, Scotland, November 7-9, 2018.

161. Shoji H, Teramoto A, Suzuki D, et al. Suture-button fixation and anterior inferior tibiofibular ligament augmentation with suture-tape for syndesmosis injury: a biomechanical cadaveric study. Clin Biomech 2018;60:121–6.

162. Teramoto A, Shoji H, Sakakibara Y, et al. Suture-button fixation and mini-open anterior inferior tibiofibular ligament augmentation using suture tape for tibiofibular syndesmosis injuries. J Foot Ankle Surg 2018;57(1):159–61.

163. Hajewski CJ, Duchman K, Goetz J, et al. Anatomic syndesmotic and deltoid ligament reconstruction with flexible implants: a technique description. Iowa Orthop J 2019;39(1):21–7.

164. Willegger M, Benca E, Hirtler L, et al. Biomechanical stability of tape augmentation for anterior talofibular ligament (ATFL) repair compared to the native ATFL. Knee Surg Sports Traumatol Arthrosc 2016. https://doi.org/10.1007/s00167-016-4048-7.

165. Yoo JS, Yang EA. Clinical results of an arthroscopic modified Brostrom operation with and without an internal brace. J Orthop Traumatol 2016. https://doi.org/10.1007/s10195-016-0406-y.

166. Cho BK, Park KJ, Park JK, et al. Outcomes of the modified Broström procedure augmented with suture-tape for ankle instability in patients with generalized ligamentous laxity. Foot Ankle Int 2017. https://doi.org/10.1177/1071100716683348.

167. Cho BK, Kim YM, Choi SM, et al. Revision anatomical reconstruction of the lateral ligaments of the ankle augmented with suture tape for patients with a failed Broström procedure. Bone Joint J 2017. https://doi.org/10.1302/0301-620X.99B9.BJJ-2017-0144.R1.

168. Coetzee JC, Ellington JK, Ronan JA, et al. Functional results of open Broström ankle ligament repair augmented with a suture tape. Foot Ankle Int 2018. https://doi.org/10.1177/1071100717742363.

169. Vega J, Montesinos E, Malagelada F, et al. Arthroscopic all-inside anterior talofibular ligament repair with suture augmentation gives excellent results in case of poor ligament tissue remnant quality. Knee Surg Sports Traumatol Arthrosc 2018;28(1):100–7.

170. DeVries JG, Scharer BM, Romdenne TA. Ankle stabilization with arthroscopic versus open with suture tape augmentation techniques. J Foot Ankle Surg 2019. https://doi.org/10.1053/j.jfas.2018.08.011.

171. Porter M, Shadbolt B, Ye X, et al. Ankle lateral ligament augmentation versus the modified Broström-Gould procedure: a 5-year randomized controlled Trial. Am J Sports Med 2019. https://doi.org/10.1177/0363546518820529.

172. Lubowitz JH, MacKay G, Gilmer B. Knee medial collateral ligament and posteromedial corner anatomic repair with internal bracing. Arthrosc Tech 2014;3(4):e505–8.

173. Peña FA, Coetzee JC. Ankle syndesmosis injuries. Foot Ankle Clin 2006;11(1):35–50.

174. Olson KM, Dairyko GH, Toolan BC. Salvage of chronic instability of the syndesmosis with distal tibiofibular arthrodesis: functional and radiographic results. J Bone Joint Surg Am 2011;93(1):66–72.

175. Katznelson A, Lin E, Militiano J. Ruptures of the ligaments about the tibio-fibular syndesmosis. Injury 1983;15(3):170–2.

176. Jeong BO, Baek JH, Song WJ. Ankle arthritis combined with chronic instability of the syndesmosis after ankle fracture with syndesmotic injury: a case report. J Foot Ankle Surg 2018;57(5):1000–4.

177. Lui TH. Arthroscopic arthrodesis of the distal tibiofibular syndesmosis. J Foot Ankle Surg 2015. https://doi.org/10.1053/j.jfas.2015.02.017.

178. Lui TH. Endoscopic distal tibiofibular syndesmosis Arthrodesis. Arthrosc Tech 2016. https://doi.org/10.1016/j.eats.2016.01.021.

Low-Energy Lisfranc Injuries
When to Fix and When to Fuse

Milap S. Patel, DO[a], Muhammad Y. Mutawakkil, MD[a],
Anish R. Kadakia, MD[b],*

KEYWORDS

- Lisfranc • Midfoot • Arthrodesis • Tarsometatarsal • Athlete

KEY POINTS

- A high index of suspicion for a Lisfranc injury is required when evaluating a patient with an injury to the midfoot.
- Stress positive and second tarsometatarsal subluxation on injury films without dorsal displacement may be treated with open reduction with internal fixation.
- Sagittal instability or the presence of articular comminution of the midfoot is better suited to an arthrodesis to ensure midfoot stability.
- Preservation of first tarsometatarsal mobility may improve the ability of the athlete to perform cutting sports.

Lisfranc injuries have classically been associated with high-energy injuries, such as from motor vehicle collisions or industrial setting accidents. High-energy injuries tend to have bony involvement with multiple fracture sites with obvious radiographic displacement. Lisfranc injuries from low-energy injuries such as from recreational or elite athletic accidents were understood to a lesser extent. Previously, low-energy athletic injuries were lightheartedly dismissed as midfoot sprains with very little consideration to the long-term consequences. However, more recently, there has been a shift in the understanding of Lisfranc injuries. Lisfranc injuries are being understood as a spectrum of injury to the Lisfranc ligament complex, which can result in variation of injury patterns.[1] In contrast with high-energy injuries, low-energy injuries are ligamentous primarily. They can vary from partial sprains with no displacement to complete tear of the Lisfranc ligament with frank diastasis.

[a] Department of Orthopedic Surgery, Northwestern Memorial Hospital, Center for Comprehensive Orthopaedic and Spine Care, 259 East Erie, 13th Floor, Chicago, IL 60611, USA;
[b] Orthopaedic Foot and Ankle Fellowship, Department of Orthopedic Surgery, Northwestern Memorial Hospital, Center for Comprehensive Orthopaedic and Spine Care, Northwestern University, 259 East Erie, 13th Floor, Chicago, IL 60611, USA
* Corresponding author.
E-mail address: Kadak259@gmail.com

Clin Sports Med 39 (2020) 773–791
https://doi.org/10.1016/j.csm.2020.07.001
0278-5919/20/© 2020 Elsevier Inc. All rights reserved.

Previously, the incidence has been reported to be 1 in 55,000 persons per year or 0.2% of all fractures.[2–4] Along with increased awareness of these injuries through education and increased use of weight-bearing radiographs, stress fluoroscopy, computed tomography (CT) scan, and MRI, the incidence of these injuries has increased.[5] With increased awareness of this injury, the incidence increased to 2.6 in 100,000 persons per year based on conventional radiographic evaluation.[6] In a recent study, with implementation of CT scan, the incidence of Lisfranc injury increased to 9.2 in 100,000 persons per year.[7]

Traditionally, Lisfranc injuries are thought of as occurring from high-energy injuries. Lievers and colleagues[8] conducted a literature review of Lisfranc dislocations in 2012 and demonstrated 43% were from traffic accidents, 24% from a fall from a height, and 13% from direct crush injury. Meanwhile, only 10% were from sport-related activities. In 2019, Ponkilainen and colleagues[7] reported 12% of injuries from traffic accidents, 16% from direct crush injury, 37% from a low-energy mechanism such as tumbling or slipping, and 9% from sport-related activities. Several other studies have also demonstrated increased percentage of injuries from low-energy mechanisms.[5,9] Again, owing to increased awareness and the use of advanced imaging, the incidence of low-energy injuries to Lisfranc complex is increasing.[6,7] Low-energy injuries account for approximately one-third of all Lisfranc injuries and occur up to 4% of National Football League players per season.[10–12] Twenty-nine percent of these injuries occur in offensive linemen.[11]

Lisfranc injuries can cause significant disability and frustration; therefore, an appropriate diagnosis and optimizing treatment is important to decrease morbidity for these patients. Low-energy injuries are often missed or misdiagnosed on initial examination owing to difficulty in diagnosis. It has been estimated that between 20% and 24% of injuries are often missed.[13–17] Therefore, a high index of suspicion is required to appropriately diagnose this injury to avoid late sequelae of post-traumatic arthrosis to midfoot, pain, decreased function, and loss of quality of life. Despite appropriate identification, there is controversy regarding what is the most effective method of treatment for these injuries. We review the treatment options and attempt to provide a logical approach to treatment of low-energy injuries, ranging from percutaneous fixation, open reduction and internal fixation (ORIF), arthrodesis, as well as novel approaches, including flexible fixation with the Internal Brace (Arthrex, Naples, FL).

ANATOMY

The tarsometatarsal (TMT) joint complex represents a transition point between the forefoot and midfoot. It is composed of multiple unique bony and ligamentous structures that provide structural support for the transverse arch.[18] There are a total of 5 metatarsals (MT) with the medial 3 metatarsals articulating with their respective cuneiform and the lateral 2 metatarsals articulating with the cuboid. The first through third MT bases, along with their respective cuneiforms, are trapezoidal shaped. The middle cuneiform is recessed proximally compared with the medial cuneiform by 8 mm and the lateral cuneiform by 4 mm, which effectively brings the second TMT joint articulation much more proximal compared with neighboring TMT joints.[19] This allows the second MT to articulate with 4 other surrounding bones besides the middle cuneiform: first MT base, medial cuneiform, third MT, and the lateral cuneiform. Owing to its unique trapezoidal shape and location, the second MT base acts as a keystone forming a stable arch known as transverse or Roman arch. The second MT is located at the apex of the midfoot, essentially wedging itself into a tightly packed location, which locks the surrounding bones into position and provides some bony stability. Peicha and colleagues[20] retrospectively compared radiographs of 33 patients with TMT joint injuries occurring from sport-related activities with cadavers with an intact Lisfranc ligament. The depth of the second MT base in relation to first TMT on anteroposterior radiograph was analyzed and it was determined that injured patients had shallower depth (8.95 mm) compared with cadaveric controls (11.61 mm).[20] Similar findings were also reported by Yu-kai and Shiu-Bii.[21] This may theoretically signify that patients with shallower second MT depth may have narrower Lisfranc ligament attachments[22] and less inherent osseous stability, which can lead to a higher rate of injury.

During the stance phase, the TMT joints are aligned perpendicular to the ground and osseous anatomy provides little inherent stability in isolation. In addition to its inherent osseous stability, the TMT joints are further stabilized by multiple soft tissues and ligamentous complex to maintain appropriate alignment and articular contact when weight bearing. The second through fifth MT bases are stabilized to each other by interosseous ligaments. There is no direct ligamentous connection between the first and second MT bases. Instead, an interosseous ligament courses obliquely from the medial cuneiform to the second MT base known as the Lisfranc ligament, which plays a crucial role in stabilizing the first ray to the rest of the midfoot. It courses from the lateral aspect of the medial cuneiform to the medial aspect of second MT base. There are other dorsal and plantar attachments between the medial cuneiform and second MT base, but they are generally weaker when compared with the plantar Lisfranc ligament.[18,22] Plantarly, the ligament originates from the lateral surface of the medial cuneiform and consists of 2 strong bands, namely, the superficial band that attaches to the third MT base and the deep band that attaches to the second MT base. In addition to these direct ligamentous structures, additional support is indirectly provided by other soft tissue structures in the plantar midfoot, including the peroneus longus tendon, long plantar ligament, the plantar fascia, and intrinsic muscles.[12,19,23] Kaar and colleagues[23] performed a cadaveric study to determine pattern of midfoot instability after sequential sectioning Lisfranc ligament complex through simulated stress radiographs. Transverse instability was observed after sectioning of interosseous Lisfranc ligament and plantar ligament. Longitudinal instability was observed after sectioning of interosseous Lisfranc ligament and intercuneiform ligaments.[23]

The midfoot can also be described as being arranged in 3 columns. The medial column is composed of navicular, medial cuneiform, and the first MT. The middle column is composed of second and third MTs along with their respective cuneiform. The lateral column is composed of fourth and fifth MTs along with its articulation with the cuboid. Owing to its mortise fit and dense ligamentous connections, the medial and middle column TMT joints have very minimal arc of motion in plantarflexion and dorsiflexion. The first TMT has a 3.5° arc of motion, the second has 0.6°, and the third has 1.6°. In contrast, the fourth has 9.6° and the fifth has 10.2°.[24] The first through third MT have nominal arc of motion when compared with fourth and fifth. The medial and the middle column are the most rigid and effectively act as a lever arm during gait while experiencing largest forces during the heel rise phase of gait. Therefore, the medial 3 TMT joints are less able to tolerate subtle instabilities, which can result from low-energy injuries compared with the relatively more mobile fourth and fifth TMT joints. Fracture or avulsion of bone at this complex results in the inherent instability of the Lisfranc complex. However, isolated ligamentous injuries can occur and also lead to similar instability. Our treatment algorithm is based on this biomechanical understanding of the motion of the midfoot, where middle column stability is critical, lateral column motion must be maintained, and, ideally, preservation of the medial column mobility may allow for superior cutting ability in sports.

MECHANISM OF INJURY

Injuries to the TMT joints can occur from either direct or indirect injuries. Direct injuries are usually from high-energy mechanisms such as a crush-type of injury. These are associated with soft tissue and/or vascular compromise. Indirect injuries are typically from low-energy mechanisms, such as from twisting of the foot. These injuries have a very subtle presentation. Renninger and colleagues[9] reported a difference between low-energy and high-energy injuries. Low-energy injuries included athletic activity, ground-level twisting, and falls from less than 4 feet. High-energy injuries included motor vehicle collisions, motorcycle collisions, direct crush, and falls from more than 4 feet.[9]

Midfoot sprains are most commonly sustained during contact sports; however, athletes involved in noncontact sports are also subject to this injury. The most common injury to the foot in athletes is trauma to the metatarsophalangeal joint followed by midfoot sprains. Midfoot sprains occurs in 4% of football players per year, with offensive linemen being the most common type of players to sustain this type of injury.[11] Shapiro and colleagues[25] described this injury in football players while the foot is plantarflexed with the metatarsophalangeal joint maximally dorsiflexed, another player falling onto the heel, which applies axial force to the foot resulting in hyperplantarflexion injury to the Lisfranc complex. Other patterns of injury have been described when forceful abduction and twisting of the foot occurs while an axial load is applied to the plantar flexed foot.[26,27] In baseball, this mechanism can occur when a player slides into a fixed base. The injury can also occur when landing onto a plantarflexed foot while parachuting.[28]

Depending on the location and amount of force applied to the TMT joints, the TMT can subluxate or dislocate in varying patterns. As discussed elsewhere in this article, the planter ligaments are stronger; therefore, dorsal displacement is more common. Less frequently, the force of injury can extend proximally through the intercuneiform joint between the medial and middle cuneiform and exit medially through the navicular-medial cuneiform joint. This injury pattern is very subtle and can lead to a significant increase in post-traumatic arthrosis if missed or managed improperly.[29,30]

Multiple classification systems have been developed in an attempt to easily identify injury pattern and guide treatment. Quenu and Kuss[31] initially described these injuries based on the direction of the MT displacement into homolateral, isolated, or divergent. Hardcastle and associates[2] modified this system into type A, B, or C based on displacement and incongruity. The most commonly used classification was described by Myerson,[12] who further modified this system based on the direction of the dislocation. Even though this classification system has a high degree of interobserver reliability, it does not guide treatment and cannot be used reliably to predict clinical results.[32] These classification systems are mainly for high-energy injuries where there are obvious radiographic changes.

Nunley and Vertullo[1] classified low-energy Lisfranc injuries sustained during sporting activities. This system guides treatment based on clinical findings, comparative weight-bearing radiographs, and bone scans. Stage I represents dorsal capsular tear without elongation of Lisfranc ligament. There is no measurable diastasis between medial cuneiform and second MT base or loss of arch height on weight-bearing radiographs, but a bone scan will demonstrate increased uptake. This type of injury can be treated nonoperatively. Stage II represents disruption of the Lisfranc ligament without injury to the plantar structures. There is diastasis between the medial cuneiform and second MT base without loss of arch height. Stage III constitutes rupture of the Lisfranc ligament with damage to the plantar ligaments, resulting in both diastasis and loss of longitudinal arch height. Stage II and III injuries should be treated surgically, as illustrated in **Table 1**. This classification helps to determine when surgical intervention is appropriate; however, it still does not help to guide what particular treatment method is ideal. Unfortunately, there are insufficient data to determine the most effective treatment method for these injuries; however, what is clearly noted is that nonsurgical management of an unstable Lisfranc injury has a greater chance of long-term morbidity than surgical stabilization or fusion.

DIAGNOSIS

The clinical history and physical examination are the most important aspects in the identification of low-energy Lisfranc injuries. In the more common mechanism, the plantar flexed position of the foot places the weaker dorsal ligamentous restraints on tension, resulting in their failure and allowing further displacement and rupture of the plantar ligamentous restraints or MT base fracture.[10,20,24] This type of injury may not produce the obvious clinical picture associated with direct high-energy injuries of severe swelling, deformity, inability to bear weight, and neurovascular compromise.[5,21] The typical presentation includes swelling throughout the midfoot that improves after 1 week and, therefore, delayed presentations may not seem to be clinically significant on visual examination.[12] Plantar ecchymosis without evidence of MT fracture or other bony injury is highly suggestive of an unstable Lisfranc injury. Persistent pain and tenderness across the midfoot that is aggravated with stress testing of the TMT joints is indicative of this injury pattern.[2] A high clinical suspicion is required in any athlete that suffered a "foot sprain" and a Lisfranc injury should be suspected until proven otherwise. High-energy mechanisms tend to have bony involvement whereas low-energy mechanisms are predominantly ligamentous, with the possibility of avulsions fractures between the medial cuneiform and the second MT base known as a fleck sign.[15]

Radiographic Evaluation

The radiographic series for a suspected Lisfranc injury should include anteroposterior, lateral, and 30° internal oblique views of both feet. Additionally, external oblique views in both 10° and 20° have demonstrated efficacy in delineating the amount of displacement in the transverse plane.[2] To stress the midfoot and demonstrate the injury radiographically, the radiographs should be performed with as much weight bearing as

Table 1
Nunley and Vertullo classification

Stage	Description	Radiographic Findings (Weight Bearing)	Treatment
I	Dorsal capsular tear without elongation of Lisfranc ligament.	No diastasis between MC and second MT base.	Cast/boot immobilization
II	Disruption of the Lisfranc ligament. Plantar structures intact.	Diastasis present between MC and second MT. No loss of arch height.	Surgical intervention
III	Rupture of the Lisfranc and plantar ligaments	Diastasis and loss of arch height	

Abbreviation: MC, medial cuneiform.

possible. Occasionally, initial weight bearing is too difficult for the patient. Therefore, if the non–weight-bearing radiographic results are normal, repeat weight-bearing views should be performed at 10 to 14 days.[20] Stress radiographs can be performed to diagnose the instability; however, they should be performed under anesthesia to prevent a false-negative finding. If possible, an ankle block can be done in the office with subsequent radiographic stress examination to minimize the morbidity of requiring sedation and minimizing the cost to the patient. The foot is stressed with pronation combined with abduction to detect subtle diastasis or angulation.[19–21] Coss and colleagues[33] have shown in a cadaveric model that disruption of the dorsal and Lisfranc ligamentous restraints resulted in a radiographic instability pattern consistently noted on abduction stress examination, verifying the usefulness of the clinical examination. The anatomic relationships of the TMT joints have consistent radiographic appearances, and deviations from these patterns are consistent with injury.[14] The medial border of the second MT is colinear with the medial border of the middle cuneiform on the anteroposterior radiographic examination along with the first intermetatarsal space and the space between the medial and middle cuneiforms. The lateral border of the third MT is colinear with the lateral border of the lateral cuneiform on the internal oblique radiograph. In addition, the medial border of the fourth MT is colinear with the medial border of the cuboid. Subtle radiographic findings include minor angulation or displacement of the first MT. Myerson and colleagues[15] described the "fleck sign," a small avulsion fracture of either the medial cuneiform or the base of the second MT, which is diagnostic of a Lisfranc disruption. Careful review of the radiographs should be performed so that Lisfranc variants with intercuneiform instability are not overlooked. In cases where the weight-bearing radiographs are negative despite a high degree of clinical suspicion, the use of an MRI is reasonable to determine the integrity of the Lisfranc ligament. If the Lisfranc ligament is not identifiable, this may indicate an unstable injury pattern, which will warrant an examination under anesthesia to determine the extent of instability and need for surgical stabilization. The use of a CT scan is considered in the setting of bony injury, where further determination of the extent of articular involvement is required to determine whether a fusion or ORIF would be appropriate. The emergence of weight-bearing CT may allow identification of subtle injuries and can be considered if weight-bearing radiographs are negative. There is no significant body of literature to determine the usefulness of weight-bearing CT scans for Lisfranc injuries and, therefore, they should not supplant weight-bearing radiographs and MRI at this time.

AUTHORS' PREFERRED TREATMENT

There is no current consensus as to the optimal treatment method for unstable Lisfranc injuries. We believe the Nunley and Vertullo's classification is a useful method by which to break down the different treatment options. We provide a detailed discussion our algorithm for treatment based on the Nunley and Vertullo classification. This algorithm is simplified in **Table 2**.

Nunley and Vertullo stage I injuries do not require surgical stabilization; however, a period of immobilization and restricted weight bearing is required. As discussed elsewhere in this article, the diagnosis is one of exclusion of instability in patients who have a clinical history of a midfoot injury. Weight-bearing radiographs must be within normal radiographic parameters and symmetric to the contralateral foot. Obtaining a single limb weight-bearing radiograph of the affected limb may improve the ability to discern subtle instability. Before initiating nonsurgical management, we currently perform an MRI of the hindfoot/midfoot to verify the integrity of the ligament. Upon verification

Table 2
Authors' treatment algorithm

Stage	Criteria	Treatment
I	MRI with evidence of Lisfranc sprain, negative stress	Cast/boot immobilization
II	Stress positive	Retrograde Lisfranc screw or suture tape fixation
	Subtle second TMT diastasis or bony Lisfranc	ORIF second TMT with plate and retrograde Lisfranc screw
	Articular comminution or significant second TMT diastasis	Arthrodesis and retrograde Lisfranc Screw
III	No first TMT articular comminution	Second/ third TMT arthrodesis with ORIF first TMT (plate or suture tape)
	First TMT articular comminution	1, 2, 3 TMT fusion

Abbreviation: TMT, tarsometatarsal joint.

of the integrity of the Lisfranc ligament with stable weight-bearing radiographs, the patient may be placed into a controlled ankle motion (CAM) walker to mechanically stabilize the midfoot and provide symptomatic relief for 6 weeks. Non–weight-bearing physical therapy with the use of bands and a stationary bike with the use of carbon fiber plate may be used to maintain muscle mass. At 6 weeks, if the patient has painless single limb weight bearing along with a painless midfoot stress examination to abduction/adduction, progression to an athletic shoe with a full-length carbon fiber plate is initiated. Physical therapy is used to gradually progress weight bearing as tolerated with the use of a gravity assist treadmill to minimize excessive stress to the midfoot. In most cases, the athlete may return to play safely at 3 months or when he or she is able to run without gravity assist. The use of a custom orthotic with carbon fiber plate within their shoes is recommended for an additional 3 months.

Nunley stage II injuries require surgical intervention to restore stability to the midfoot. In these cases, by definition, there is no sagittal instability and surgical treatment needs to only restore coronal stability. We divide these patients into 2 categories for the purpose of determining the appropriate procedure. In patients who have a stress positive only instability of the second TMT, we consider either a percutaneous screw placed retrograde or the use of a suture tape construct.[34–36] There is clearly controversy when discussing percutaneous fixation for Lisfranc injuries and the surgeon must weigh the benefit of a minimally invasive approach versus a traditional open approach. We feel that when diastasis is present only under stress testing, and alignment is symmetric to the uninjured lower extremity, percutaneous fixation may allow for stabilization without a formal open approach. A reduction clamp is used in this technique to ensure appropriate alignment during fixation (**Fig. 1**). Alternatively, a longitudinal incision made just medial to the third TMT joint allows for excellent access to the lateral second MT and the Lisfranc articulation while minimizing the risk to the deep peroneal nerve and the first dorsal interosseous artery. A large reduction clamp should be used as well to ensure a stable reduction of the joint. To facilitate placement of the screw, we use a cannulated drill followed by a solid 3.5-mm screw. Based on our experience, we have found that a retrograde Lisfranc screw minimizes risk of injury to the anterior tibial tendon and maximizes bony purchase in the second MT.

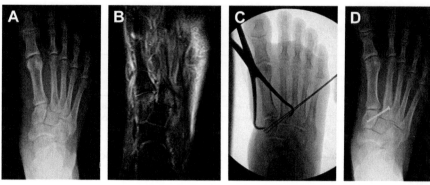

Fig. 1. Preoperative non–weight-bearing radiograph of a patient with a suspected Lisfranc injury (*A*). MRI demonstrated disruption of the Lisfranc ligament noted by an inability to visualize any ligamentous tissue between the medial cuneiform and base of the second MT. The bony edema of noted in both the medial cuneiform and second MT is also indicative of injury (*B*). Percutaneous reduction and stabilization with a large tenaculum followed by retrograde guidewire placement (*C*). The starting position of the screw is approximately 1 cm distal to the second MT. Postoperative appearance at 1 year demonstrates stable alignment without hardware failure (*D*).

For patients who have a subtle diastasis on non–weight-bearing injuries without involvement of the first TMT or those with a large bony proximal fragment without articular comminution ("bony Lisfranc"), we perform an open reduction with a transarticular plate and retrograde Lisfranc screw as discussed elsewhere in this article. In the setting of either a significantly displaced ligamentous injury or articular comminution, we prefer an arthrodesis of the second and/or third TMT joint in association with a retrograde Lisfranc screw. There is a significant controversy as to whether this injury should be treated with arthrodesis or ORIF. We have performed both methods of treatment for this injury and our results are consistent with recent literature.[37–39] Our experience is that we are able to achieve more reproducible results with an arthrodesis with a decreased rate of subsequent surgery. However, in subtle cases of second TMT malalignment we do perform ORIF without hardware removal because this technique provides stability while minimizing the risk of recurrent displacement (**Fig. 2**). The term "closet fuser" has been used to describe this type of protocol. We do not feel routine hardware removal is necessary based on the concept that the middle column serves to provide midfoot stability, with minimal motion at the second and third TMT joints.

The surgical approach is similar as discussed elsewhere in this article, because this allows facile exposure of both the second and third TMT joints. Note that this incision is more lateral than the more commonly described first webspace–based incision and does not allow exposure of the first TMT. Standard joint preparation is performed with the use of osteotomes and curettes, with subchondral drilling after articular cartilage removal. Although the use of a saw may be considered, this method does increase the risk of excessive bone resection with a subsequent inability to compress the joint and, therefore, is not our preferred method of choice. Autograft or allograft may be placed in the arthrodesis based on surgeon preference, but is not required if good bone on bone apposition is achieved. In the setting of an isolated second TMT arthrodesis, the intermetatarsal ligament between the proximal second and third MTs should be released to allow for mobility of the second MT so bone-on-bone apposition may occur. Fixation is performed with a transarticular compression plate. We prefer this method of fixation given the reproducible nature of plate fixation compared with screw

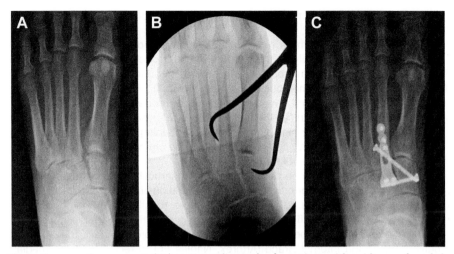

Fig. 2. Preoperative non–weight-bearing radiograph of a patient with evidence of a subtle Lisfranc injury without significant subluxation (*A*). An open approach was used to reduce the second TMT using a large tenaculum with direct visualization of the alignment (*B*). Final appearance 1 year postoperatively following transarticular plating and placement of a retrograde Lisfranc screw with additional intercuneiform fixation that is stable without hardware failure (*C*). Intercuneiform fixation is not required when using transarticular second TMT plating with an additional Lisfranc screw because intercuneiform stability is indirectly achieved in these cases. However, when using only screw fixation for these injuries that are clear on non–weight-bearing radiographs, we routinely use intercuneiform fixation to ensure medial to middle column stability.

fixation. The ultimate method of fixation is not as critical as long as rigid stability is achieved. In all cases we use a retrograde Lisfranc screw to ensure stability.

Given the minimal motion at the second TMT articulation and the importance of stability over motion for this joint, we no longer routinely perform hardware removal for this type of injury. Although the screw may fatigue with progressive activity, given the lack of sagittal instability, we have not found this issue to be significant clinically. If the patient or surgeon has concern about this complication, we advocate delayed hardware removal at 4 to 5 months from surgery to ensure adequate ligamentous healing has occurred.

Nunley type 3 injuries are more high-energy and typically involve the first, second, and third TMT joints and in some cases the fourth and fifth as well. Both sagittal and coronal instability is present in this situation with a higher failure rate of ORIF in these cases. In the setting of dorsal displacement indicating complete ligamentous instability, the consensus is largely that arthrodesis is the most reliable method of treatment of both the medial and middle columns. Transarticular pinning with removal of hardware at 5 to 6 weeks for the lateral column is performed if required. However, based on the biomechanics of the medial column, there is relevant motion present that is eliminated after arthrodesis of the first TMT that may affect high-level athletic play. In some of our patients after first TMT arthrodesis and with discussion with colleagues, there are anecdotal complaints of persistent first ray overload and pain within the sesamoids with impact or running activity. This pain is difficult to mitigate despite the use of orthotics and may compromise high-level athletic performance. Unfortunately, there is no current literature to compare ORIF of the first TMT with arthrodesis of the first TMT in the setting of a Lisfranc injury where the second and third TMT have been fused.

We have a novel algorithm for high-level athletes when dealing with this complex injury pattern, based primarily on the concept that arthrodesis of the middle column imparts rigid stability to the midfoot and eliminates the abduction instability of the first TMT. In the setting of a ligamentous injury to the first TMT without articular comminution, we prefer ORIF of the first TMT combined with arthrodesis of the middle column. We believe this hybrid fixation can the restore stability of the midfoot while maintaining relevant first TMT motion for high-level activity. Maintaining the supination/pronation function of the midfoot during cutting activity may be critical for a high level athlete to return to the preinjury level of function.

ORIF of the first TMT can be performed with transarticular plating that should be removed at 4 months postoperatively, before the initiation of gravity-assisted physical therapy. Although hardware removal should restore mobility of the joint, we have noted that significant joint stiffness can persist, along with irritation of the anterior tibial tendon secondary to irritation from the hardware. Therefore, we have used a novel technique using the Internal Brace (Arthrex, Naples FL) to reconstruct the medial/plantar first TMT capsuloligamentous complex combined with arthrodesis of the middle column. Our preferred approach is a medial incision centered over the first TMT. This method does require the use of 2 incisions as opposed to a single dorsal first webspace incision; however, we have not found this to increase the risk of wound complications. Additionally, the visualization of the first TMT, specifically the plantar aspect, is easily made through a medial approach as opposed to a dorsal approach. The use of the suture tape/interference screw construct is a novel concept and we have performed this method on 5 patients with excellent clinical outcomes; however, we do emphasize that this technique is relatively new without long-term follow-up.

Both the dorsal incision immediately medial to the third MT and the medial first TMT incision is made. Reduction and final fixation of the middle column is performed before placement of the suture tape construct. To prevent over-reduction of the second TMT, a 0.062-inch K-wire may be placed across the first TMT to maintain the position before fixation of the middle column. The initial fixation point is along the plantar medial aspect of the proximal first MT (**Fig. 3**). The suture tape is then taken proximal and secured to the distal medial cuneiform, taking care to ensure that there is no irritation of the anterior tibial tendon (**Fig. 4**). The tape has a low profile, allowing the cuneiform fixation to be placed deep to the tendon with minimal risk of irritation to the tendon.

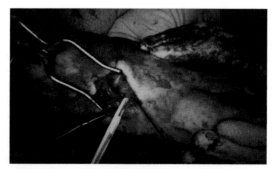

Fig. 3. The initial fixation point of the suture tape is along the plantar medial aspect of the first MT. Note the angle of the insertion device as it is angle superiorly to ensure placement within the MT and avoid perforation of the plantar cortex.

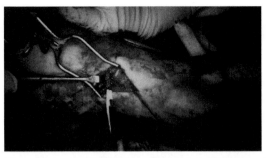

Fig. 4. After retraction of the anterior tibial tendon and stabilization of the reduced first TMT (performed with a K-wire), the proximal fixation within the medial cuneiform is completed. With placement a K-wire we secure the proximal screw with the suture tape under tension as it is not possible to over-reduce the joint in this case.

Tensioning can be difficult and although the use of a K-wire simplifies this issue, some surgeons may not be comfortable with the minimal articular injury that occurs. Alternatively, an assistant can hold the first TMT reduced by dorsiflexing the first MTP as this aids in reduction, while the surgeon performs proximal fixation with the interference screw. Excess suture tape is cut leaving a low profile construct that is flush to the bone (**Fig. 5**). In combination with a middle column fusion, we have found this construct to be excellent for restoration of first TMT stability while minimizing damage to the joint; it mitigates the need for a second surgery to remove the hardware. We have performed this technique on a Division I football player who suffered a devastating 1 through 5 Lisfranc fracture/dislocation (**Fig. 6**). He has been able to return to full athletic play as a starting quarterback at 9 months postoperatively with anatomic alignment (**Fig. 7**). We feel preservation of some of the first TMT mobility has allowed him to maintain this high level of agility.

A variant that does not fit well into any particular classification system is the intercuneiform variant. This injury is frequently misdiagnosed because there is minimal to no malalignment of the second TMT. To identify this naviculocuneiform variant, a high index of suspicion is required with a focus on the distal navicular and intercuneiform

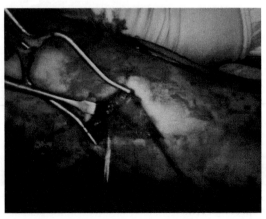

Fig. 5. Final appearance of the construct before cutting the excess suture tape. The plantar medial placement of the device can be seen.

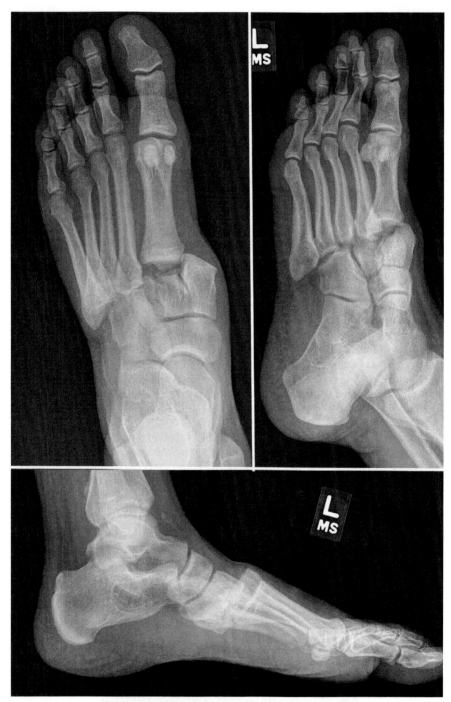

Fig. 6. Injury films of a collegiate football player who suffered a 1 through Lisfranc fracture/dislocation during a sporting event.

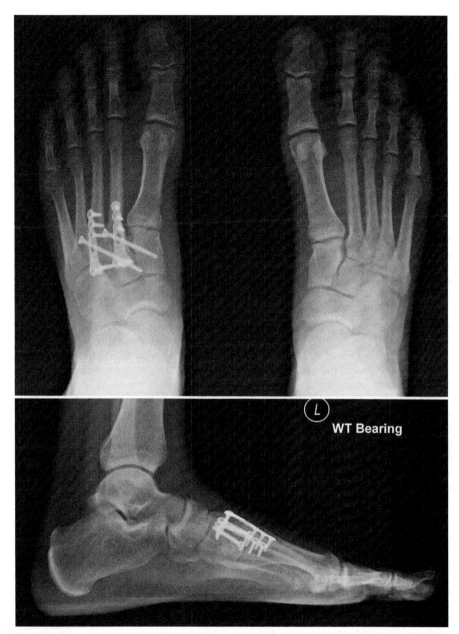

Fig. 7. Radiographic appearance 9 months postoperative of the athlete in **Fig. 6** noting symmetric alignment of the affected left foot compared with the right. Successful arthrodesis was achieved of the second and third TMT with closed reduction of the fourth and fifth TMT. Note the reduced position of the first TMT on both the anteroposterior and lateral radiographs with the suture tape construct.

diastasis that should be compared with the contralateral lower extremity if there is any equivocation of the diagnosis. A subtle fracture of the distal medial navicular is a sign that loss of stability of the medial column has occurred (**Fig. 8**). Failure to stabilize the intercuneiform joint will result in failure of fixation secondary to proximal migration of the medial column. An open approach with a first web space–based incision is advocated in this variant to ensure adequate exposure. The first MT must be distracted with direct visualization of the naviculocuneiform joint to improve the accuracy of an anatomic reduction. Initial K-wire fixation is placed from the medial to middle/lateral cuneiform to ensure length stability. The second MT may then be reduced to the now stable and anatomically aligned medial column and fixated. If an arthrodesis is considered, joint preparation is performed between the medial and middle cuneiform as well as the second TMT if unstable. Fixation for the intercuneiform joint can be performed either with a screw or dorsally placed compression staple. In all cases, a retrograde Lisfranc screw is placed. In this unique setting, the intercuneiform fixation is required and we do not perform hardware removal in these cases because stability is more relevant than the minimal motion between the medial and middle cuneiform (**Fig. 9**).

Postoperative recovery for all surgical fixation is similar to ensure appropriate ligamentous healing/arthrodesis. A splint is placed immediately postoperatively and left for 2 weeks. At 2 weeks, the patient may be placed into a CAM boot for gentle range of motion exercises. However, non–weight bearing is maintained for another 4 weeks. Non–weight-bearing physical therapy with the use of bands along with edema control is initiated. At 6 weeks, if the patient has minimal pain with radiographs consistent with anatomic alignment and appropriate healing, weight bearing is initiated with a CAM walker boot. Physical therapy is progressed to allow stationary biking with a carbon fiber plate with resistance band exercises to tolerance. At 3 months, progression to weight bearing in an athletic shoe with a full-length carbon fiber plate is initiated. Physical therapy is progressed to weight bearing as tolerated with the use of a gravity assist treadmill to minimize excessive stress to the midfoot. In most cases, the athlete may return to practice at 4.5 months or when able to run without gravity assist. Full return to play is variable based on the severity of the injury, with patients who require an arthrodesis typically requiring at least 6 months before returning to play. Full recovery to achieve a preinjury level may require 11 to 12 months. The use of a custom orthotic with carbon fiber plate within their shoes is recommended for a full year.

RESULTS

There a multitude of studies that have described the outcomes after Lisfranc injuries; however, only a limited body of literature exists when considering the elite athlete. We focus on the results that are most relevant to the athletic population.

Deol and colleagues[40] reported on the outcomes of treated 17 patients who sustained a Lisfranc injury while playing professional rugby and soccer. Ten patients had bony injury (Hardcastle B and C) and 7 had ligamentous disruption (Nunley II). Fifteen patients underwent treatment with Lisfranc screw with or without a TMT plate or screw. The remaining 2 patient underwent arthrodesis. Hardware was removed in all patients at 16 weeks. Sixteen of the 17 patients returned to training at 20.1 weeks and subsequently participated in competitive games at 25.3 weeks.[40]

McHale and colleagues[41] evaluated the effect of a Lisfranc injury on the prospects and career of the college football athletes at the National Football League Combine. They showed that this injury presents a significant adverse effect on a player's draft status, draft position, and number of games played in the first 2 years of professional

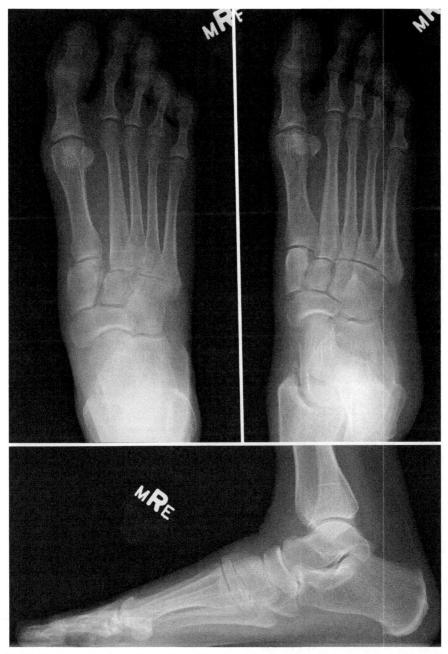

Fig. 8. Radiographs of a patient who suffered an intercuneiform Lisfranc variant with additional second TMT subluxation. Widening between the medial and middle cuneiform along with dorsal subluxation of both the first MT and medial cuneiform as a unit should alert the surgeon to this diagnosis. This finding is in distinction to the more common Lisfranc injury, where the first MT is dorsally subluxated relative to the cuneiform.

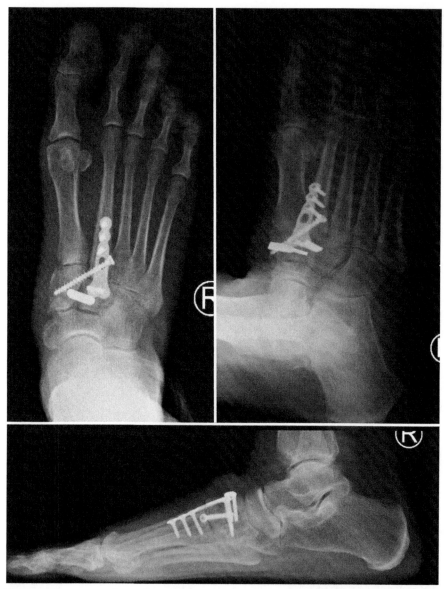

Fig. 9. Final postoperative radiographs at 1 year noting persistent stability of the reduction without failure of the hardware. The limited motion of the second TMT and the intercuneiform joints does not impart significant stress to the construct. We feel maintenance of stability with the small inherent risk of hardware failure is superior to hardware removal and risk of loss of alignment in this variant.

career. Despite this detriment attributable to the injury itself, surgical management does not eliminate the player's chances of returning to play at an elite level.[41] Singh and colleagues[42] reported about 83% rate of return to play within 10 months among National Football League players. However, they noted a significant decrease in participation and overall performance particularly in offensive players.

Cochran and colleagues[43] compared the outcomes of primary arthrodesis versus ORIF in low-energy Lisfranc injuries among young athletic patients in the military. They reported a significantly faster return to full duty among the arthrodesis group (4.5 months vs 6.7 months), as well as better fitness test scores at 1 year but found no difference between Foot and Ankle Ability Measure scores after 3 years.[43] Similarly, Henning and colleagues[44] found no difference in Medical Outcomes Short Form 36 item and Short Musculoskeletal Function Assessment scores at 2 years between arthrodesis and ORIF in treating ligamentous or combined injuries. The authors concluded that either treatment method is appropriate when done properly.[44]

SUMMARY

Lisfranc injuries represent a significant compromise to the mechanical stability of the midfoot. The most critical aspect in dealing with these injuries is identification of the injury as opposed to the nuances of the various surgical options. Persistent midfoot instability will negatively impact the ability of an athlete to play at the elite level. We have presented an algorithmic approach when approaching these difficult patterns of instability with the concept of minimizing surgical risk with a focus on middle column stability and preservation of medial column mobility. Although there are limited studies in the athletic population, they show that a majority of patients are able to preinjury activities including elite sports regardless of treatment method (ORIF vs fusion). When counseling both the professional and recreational athlete, it is critical to inform them that some patients will be unable to return to high level sports, as setting appropriate expectations is critical in this high demand patient population. Additionally, professional players should be informed about the potential effect of the injury on their performance upon return to play. A Lisfranc injury does not equivocally mean the end of an athletic career as long as the injury is recognized and midfoot stability is restored.

DISCLOSURE

Arthrex – Consultant, Speaker's Bureau.

REFERENCES

1. Nunley JA, Vertullo CJ. Classification, investigation, and management of midfoot sprains: Lisfranc injuries in the athlete. Am J Sports Med 2002;30(6):871–8.

2. Hardcastle PH, Reschauer R, Kutscha-Lissberg E, et al. Injuries to the tarsometatarsal joint: incidence, classification and treatment. J Bone Joint Surg Br 1982; 64:349–56.

3. Aitken AP, Poulson D. Dislocations of the tarsometatarsal joint. J Bone Joint Surg Am 1963;45:246–60.

4. English TA. Dislocations of the metatarsal bone and adjacent toe. J Bone Joint Surg Br 1964;46:700–4.

5. Stødle AH, Hvaal KH, Enger M, et al. Lisfranc injuries: incidence, mechanisms of injury and predictors of instability. Foot Ankle Surg 2020;26(5):535–40.

6. Vuori JP, Aro HT. Lisfranc joint injuries: trauma mechanisms and associated injuries. J Trauma 1993;35(1):40–5.

7. Ponkilainen VT, Laine HJ, Mäenpää HM, et al. Incidence and characteristics of midfoot injuries. Foot Ankle Int 2019;40(1):105–12.

8. Lievers WB, Frimenko RE, Crandall JR, et al. Age, sex, causal and injury patterns in tarsometatarsal dislocations: a literature review of over 2000 cases. Foot 2012; 22(3):117–24.

9. Renninger CH, Cochran G, Tompane T, et al. Injury characteristics of low-energy Lisfranc injuries compared with high energy injuries. Foot Ankle Int 2017;38(9): 964–9.

10. Watson TS, Shurnas PS, Denker J. Treatment of Lisfranc joint injury: current concepts. J Am Acad Orthop Surg 2010;18(12):718–28.

11. Meyer SA, Callaghan JJ, Albright JP, et al. Midfoot sprains in collegiate football players. Am J Sports Med 1994;22(3):392–401.

12. Myerson MS. The diagnosis and treatment of injury to the tarsometatarsal joint complex. J Bone Joint Surg Br 1999;81:756–63.

13. Chiodo CP, Myerson MS. Developments and advances in the diagnosis and treatment of injuries to the tarsometatarsal joint. Orthop Clin North Am 2001;32(1): 11–20.

14. Haapamaki VV, Kiuru MJ, Koskinen SK. Ankle and foot injuries: analysis of MDCT findings. AJR Am J Roentgenol 2004;183(3):615–22.

15. Myerson MS, Fisher RT, Burgess AR, et al. Fracture dislocations of the tarsometatarsal joints: end results correlated with pathology and treatment. Foot Ankle 1986;6(5):225–42.

16. Stavlas P, Roberts CS, Xypnitos FN, et al. The role of reduction and internal fixation of Lisfranc fracture-dislocations: a systematic review of the literature. Int Orthop 2010;34(8):1083–91.

17. Thompson MC, Mormino MA. Injury to the tarsometatarsal joint complex. J Am Acad Orthop Surg 2003;11(4):260–7.

18. de Palma L, Santucci A, Sabetta SP, et al. Anatomy of the Lisfranc joint complex. Foot Ankle Int 1997;18(6):356–64.

19. Sarrafian SK, Kelikian AS. Syndesmology. In: Kelikian AS, editor. Sarrafian's anatomy of the foot and ankle: descriptive, topographic, functional. Philadelphia: Lippincott; 2011. p. 208–12.

20. Peicha G, Labovitz J, Seibert FJ, et al. The anatomy of the joint as a risk factor for Lisfranc dislocation and fracture-dislocation: an anatomical and radiological case control study. J Bone Joint Surg Br 2002;84(7):981–5.

21. Yu-Kai Y, Shiu-Bii L. Anatomic parameters of the Lisfranc joint complex in a radiographic and cadaveric comparison. J Foot Ankle Surg 2015;54(5):883–7.

22. Solan MC, Moorman CT III, Miyamoto RG, et al. Ligamentous restraints of the second tarsometatarsal joint: a biomechanical evaluation. Foot Ankle Int 2001; 22(8):637–41.

23. Kaar S, Femino J, Morag Y. Lisfranc joint displacement following sequential ligament sectioning. J Bone Joint Surg Am 2007;89:2225–32.

24. Ouzounian TJ, Shereff MJ. In vitro determination of midfoot motion. Foot Ankle 1989;10(3):140–6.

25. Shapiro MS, Wascher DC, Finerman GA. Rupture of Lisfranc's ligament in athletes. Am J Sports Med 1994;22(5):687–91.

26. Harwood MI, Raikin SM. A Lisfranc fracture-dislocation in a football player. J Am Board Fam Pract 2003;16(1):69–72.

27. Wiley JJ. The mechanism of tarso-metatarsal joint injuries. J Bone Joint Surg Br 1971;53(3):474–82.

28. Curtis MJ, Myerson M, Szura B. Tarsometatarsal joint injuries in the athlete. Am J Sports Med 1993;21(4):497–502.

29. Lewis JS Jr, Anderson RB. Lisfranc injuries in the athlete. Foot Ankle Int 2016; 37(12):1374–80.
30. Myerson MS, Cerrato R. Current management of tarsometatarsal injuries in the athlete. Instr Course Lect 2009;58:583–94.
31. Quenu E, Kuss GE. Etude sur les luxations du metatarse (Luxations metatarso-tarsiennes). Du diastasis entre le 1er et le 2e metatarsien. Rev Chir 1909;39:1–72.
32. Talarico RH, Hamilton GA, Ford LA, et al. Fracture dislocations of the tarsometa-tarsal joints: analysis of interrater reliability in using the modified Hardcastle clas-sification system. J foot Ankle Surg 2006;45(5):300–3.
33. Coss HS, Manos RE, Buoncristiani A, et al. Abduction stress and AP weightbear-ing radiography of purely ligamentous injury in the tarsometatarsal joint. Foot Ankle Int 1998;19(8):537–41.
34. Panchbhavi VK, Vallurupalli S, Yang J, et al. Screw fixation compared with suture-button fixation of isolated Lisfranc ligament injuries. J Bone Joint Surg Am 2009; 91(5):1143–8.
35. Hopkins J, Heyrani N, Kreulen C, et al. Internal brace has comparable stiffness and strength as tightrope for Lisfranc fixation. J Orthop 2019;17:7–12.
36. Panchbhavi VK. Orientation of the "Lisfranc Screw". J Orthop Trauma 2012; 26(11):e221–4.
37. Seybold JD, Coetzee JC. Lisfranc injuries: when to observe, fix, or fuse. Clin Sports Med 2015;34(4):705–23.
38. Weatherford BM, Anderson JG, Bohay DR. Management of Tarsometatarsal Joint Injuries. J Am Acad Orthop Surg 2017;25(7):469–79.
39. Hawkinson MP, Tennent DJ, Belisle J, et al. Outcomes of Lisfranc injuries in an active duty military population. Foot Ankle Int 2017;38(10):1115–9.
40. Deol RS, Roche A, Calder JD. Return to training and playing after acute Lisfranc injuries in elite professional soccer and rugby players. Am J Sports Med 2016; 44(1):166–70.
41. McHale KJ, Vopat BG, Beaulieu-Jones BR, et al. Epidemiology and outcomes of Lisfranc injuries identified at the National Football League scouting combine. Am J Sports Med 2017;45(8):1901–8.
42. Singh SK, George A, Kadakia AR, et al. Performance-based outcomes following Lisfranc injury among professional American football and rugby athletes. Ortho-pedics 2018;41(4):e479–82.
43. Cochran G, Renninger C, Tompane T, et al. Primary arthrodesis versus open reduction and internal fixation for low-energy Lisfranc injuries in a young athletic population. Foot Ankle Int 2017;38(9):957–63.
44. Henning JA, Jones CB, Sietsema DL, et al. Open reduction internal fixation versus primary arthrodesis for Lisfranc injuries: a prospective randomized study. Foot Ankle Int 2009;30(10):913–22.

Cavovarus
Fifth Metatarsal Fractures and Revision Open Reduction Internal Fixation

Carroll P. Jones, MD

KEYWORDS

- Jones fracture • Recurrent Jones fracture • Cavus • Cavovarus

KEY POINTS

- Any patient that presents with a recurrent proximal fifth metatarsal (MT) fracture should be closely examined for cavovarus alignment, because it may be subtle.
- In the setting of cavovarus alignment, a recurrent zone 2/3 fifth MT fracture typically requires a revision with more robust fixation and biologics, and possibly the addition of osteotomies to address the foot deformity.
- The decision on whether or not to add a cavovarus reconstruction to the revision open reduction internal fixation is debatable and depends on several factors, notably: patient demographics, activity level, severity of deformity, and quality of index procedure. Most revisions are successfully achieved without addressing the cavovarus alignment, assuming it is mild.

INTRODUCTION

Proximal fifth metatarsal (MT) fractures have been classified by Dameron[1] into three zones based on anatomic location (**Fig. 1**). The proximal metaphysis and diaphysis are included in zones 2 and 3, respectively. Fractures in these two areas have high nonunion and refracture rates, likely related to a "watershed" of vascular insufficiency.[2,3] For the purpose of this article, zone 2 and 3 fractures are collectively called "Jones" fractures based on similarities in clinical outcomes and challenges.[4,5]

Nonoperative treatment (prolonged cast immobilization and nonweightbearing) of Jones fractures has been shown to have high failure rates. Many authors have recommended immediate surgical intervention with intramedullary screw for acute Jones fractures to provide higher union rates and quicker return to play, and this has been widely adopted as the treatment of choice for the athletic population.[6–8]

Despite more aggressive surgical strategies and improved implant strength,[9] recurrent fractures and persistent nonunions still occur, albeit at much lower rates

OrthoCarolina Foot & Ankle Institute, Atrium MSK Institute, 2001 Vail Avenue, Suite 200B, Charlotte, NC 28207, USA
E-mail address: carrolljones3@gmail.com
Twitter: @fxdoc; @ankleinstitute (C.P.J.)

Clin Sports Med 39 (2020) 793–799
https://doi.org/10.1016/j.csm.2020.07.006   **sportsmed.theclinics.com**

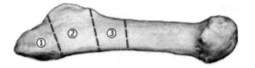

Fig. 1. Fifth metatarsal base fracture classification. Zone 1: tuberosity avulsion. Zone 2: metaphyseal fracture (classic "Jones" fracture). Zone 3: proximal diaphyseal fracture.

compared with nonoperative management. Identified risk factors for failure include small diameter and/or cannulated screws,[10] overaggressive rehabilitation,[11] inherent biologic insufficiency, and varus hindfoot.[12] This article provides guidelines for treatment of a recurrent fracture or nonunion with a concomitant cavovarus foot deformity.

CONTENT

Each patient that presents with a recurrent fracture should be carefully evaluated with attention to: (1) the implants used at the index procedure, (2) position of the implant, (3) the postoperative protocol used, (4) the metabolic status (ie, vitamin D and calcium levels), and (5) the standing posture of the foot. Any metabolic condition (ie, anorexia or vitamin D deficiency) or hormonal abnormalities (ie, amenorrhea) should undergo corrective therapy before attempted revision surgery. Referral to a nutritionist, psychologist or psychiatrist, endocrinologist, or obstetrician-gynecologist should be considered for cases that cannot be comfortably addressed by the treating orthopedist.

Raikin and colleagues,[12] in a series of 21 primary Jones fractures treated surgically, noted clinical cavus alignment in 16 (76%) feet. Even in the setting of a cavus foot, the authors demonstrated a 100% union rate with intramedullary screw fixation alone,

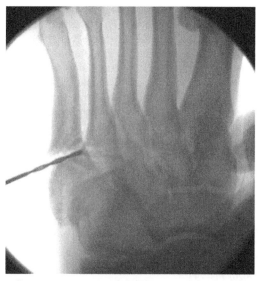

Fig. 2. Intraoperative fluoroscopic image of drill fenestration and preparation of nonunion/refracture site.

with appropriate orthotic inserts after healing had occurred. For the patient that presents with a recurrent fracture after intramedullary screw fixation and mild cavus, it is reasonable to consider intramedullary screw exchange to a larger diameter, and preferably, solid screw, with autologous bone grafting.

The technique includes an incision that is made proximal to the base of the fifth MT, ideally along the previous surgical scar. If the screw is intact, it is removed through this incision. If the screw is broken, the proximal portion is removed and the distal part of the screw is extracted with a broken-screw removal tray. Less commonly, and only if necessary, a trough is created more distally in the MT for removal of distal part of the screw. Once the screw fragments are removed, a 1- to 2-cm incision is made over the nonunion or refracture site (fluoroscopy is used for site of the incision). A periosteal flap is created sharply and reflected dorsally and plantarly to expose the fracture site. The fracture is debrided with curettes and fenestrated with a small drill (**Fig. 2**) and then packed with autologous graft. Bone marrow is aspirated from the iliac crest and concentrated and mixed with allograft, or autograft is harvested from the ilium or calcaneus.

After preparing and grafting the nonunion, a solid drill bit works well (even in reverse) to carefully create a new intramedullary path through the base of the fifth MT and into the canal. Extreme care is taken, with the assistance of fluoroscopy, to avoid penetrating a cortex. Once the correct path has been created, hand reamers are used in

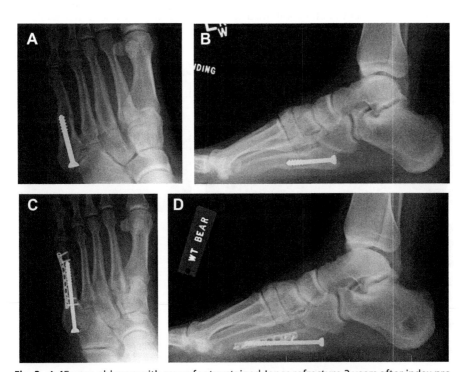

Fig. 3. A 45-year-old man with cavus foot sustained Jones refracture 3 years after index procedure. He was treated with intramedullary screw exchange, plate fixation, and calcaneal autograft. (*A*) Preoperative oblique radiograph demonstrating refracture around distal portion of screw. (*B*) Preoperative lateral radiograph highlights cavus foot alignment. (*C*, *D*) Oblique and lateral postoperative radiographs showing complete fracture union 3 months after revision.

sequentially larger diameters until the right "fit" and torque resistance is met. A partially threaded screw is then inserted, with a length allowing the threads to be just past the fracture. Long screws may overstraighten the typically curved fifth MT and actually distract the fracture. For revision cases, a solid 5.5-mm diameter screw with a 40- to 50-mm length is often the ideal size. For larger patients, a 6.5-mm screw is sometimes required to obtain adequate cortical fixation. It is important to use a system with a range of screw sizes and lengths. It should be noted that a headless screw may gain superior proximal fixation of the fifth MT, but bone loss during explant may further complicate revision fixation.

Depending on the size of the defect, 4 to 6 weeks of nonweightbearing may be necessary, followed by progressive weightbearing in a walking boot for a similar length of time. Vitamin D and calcium supplementation and use of an external bone stimulator are also recommended during the initial postoperative period. A computed tomography scan is obtained at 10 to 12 weeks to assess healing and help determine return to activity, in addition to evaluation of clinical progress. A custom orthotic to address the cavovarus alignment is fabricated and used for athletic activity, indefinitely. The prescription for the orthotic should include a recessed first ray and lateral heel posting to help correct cavovarus alignment, if flexible. Patients with rigid deformities may not be able to tolerate a corrective orthotic, and an accommodative insert may be considered.

Alternatively, plate fixation with or without intramedullary screw fixation may be used for the recurrent fracture with mild cavus. A plate may provide better torsional

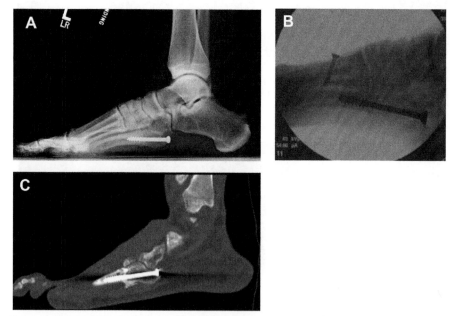

Fig. 4. Professional basketball player treated with revision screw fixation and first MT dorsiflexion osteotomy after two failed surgeries. (A) Lateral radiograph demonstrating Jones fracture nonunion and cavus foot. (B) Intraoperative fluoroscopic image of exchange screw fixation of fifth MT and first MT dorsiflexion osteotomy. (C) Three-month postoperative computed tomography scan with solid union of fifth MT revision. (Courtesy of Robert Anderson, MD.)

stability and compression, particularly if an intramedullary screw does not achieve reasonable purchase because of bone loss or defect (**Fig. 3**). Additionally, a plate is applied more plantarly and offers the biomechanical advantage of being on the tension side of the refracture.

If the patient has undergone more than one failed attempt at internal fixation and/or has a significant cavovarus foot posture, corrective osteotomies are recommended to provide a plantigrade foot and minimize the abnormal load on the fifth MT. Coleman block testing is used to identify the flexibility of the cavovarus, and whether it is fore-foot or hindfoot driven. In addition to the steps outlined previously to revise and bone graft the nonunion, the surgeon may elect to perform a first MT dorsiflexion osteotomy, a lateral closing wedge/slide calcaneal osteotomy, or in some cases, both. In the ath-letic population, extreme caution is urged before undertaking these more complex reconstructive adjunctive procedures. Healing times, the rehabilitation process, and return to play are likely to take much longer and be far less predictable. Anecdotally,

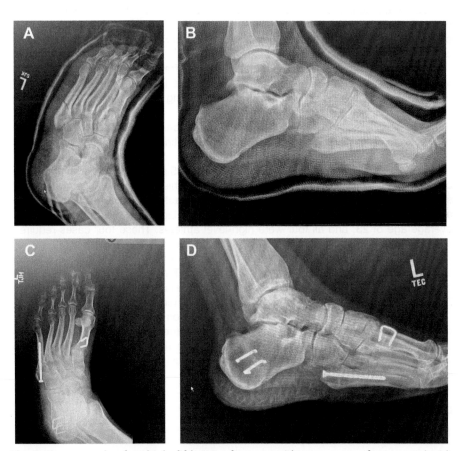

Fig. 5. Case example of multiple fifth MT refractures with severe cavus foot treated with screw fixation of MT fracture and Dwyer calcaneal and first MT osteotomies. (*A*) Oblique radiograph of recurrent Jones fracture. (*B*) Preoperative lateral radiograph of cavus foot. (*C, D*) Postoperative oblique and lateral radiographs demonstrating healed fifth MT fracture and osteotomies. (*Courtesy of* J. Randolph Clements, DPM.)

a first MT dorsiflexion osteotomy alone is often enough and is far less morbid than a calcaneal osteotomy (although minimally invasive techniques may change this).

Fig. 4 is a case example of a professional basketball player who had two previous failed attempts at fifth MT intramedullary fixation for an acute Jones fracture and underwent revision open reduction internal fixation with bone grafting, with a dorsiflexion first MT osteotomy to address cavus alignment, which was believed to be contributing to the recurrent nonunions. At 12 weeks, computed tomography scan demonstrated a solid union, and he was able to return to professional-level play.

Fig. 5 is a case example of an individual who had sustained multiple fifth MT refractures, despite casting and shoe-wear/insert modification. Although a less common scenario, because of the severe associated cavovarus deformity, this was treated successfully with intramedullary screw fixation with calcaneal and first MT osteotomies.

SUMMARY

Aggressive surgical treatment of acute Jones fractures has been shown to expedite healing and return to activity, and lower the nonunion rate.[7,8] The cavovarus foot is clearly a predisposing factor for sustaining this injury, but the decision-making to address the foot deformity is unclear and debatable.[12]

Raikin and colleagues,[12] in a series of acute Jones fractures, treated all patients (21 feet) with screw fixation alone. Despite having a 76% incidence of cavus foot alignment, 100% union was achieved without addressing the malalignment surgically. Hunt and Anderson[7] reported on the treatment of Jones fracture nonunions and refractures in the elite athlete. Although the incidence of cavus foot alignment was not reported, all patients achieved healing with grafting and revision screw fixation with full return to play, with only one refracture.

Granata and colleagues[10] reported on a series of 55 patients younger than the age of 40 with a minimum 1-year follow-up. All patients achieved union with intramedullary screw fixation but four patients (7.3%) sustained refractures. All four refractures were associated with bent, small-diameter screws (ranging from 3.5–5.0 mm) with an average age of 23, and all four were high-level athletes. These four cases required screw revision, and one also underwent a Dwyer calcaneal osteotomy.

Based on published literature, even in the setting of a cavus foot, most patients achieve high union rates with fixation of the fifth MT alone, assuming the screw is appropriately sized and positioned correctly and there is a diligent postoperative rehabilitation course. Residual varus can typically be treated with orthotic management.

However, if there is a pattern of refracture/nonunion in the setting of a significant cavovarus foot, osteotomies to restore a plantigrade foot may be necessary to create the right biomechanics for healing. This should be undertaken with considerable caution to the patient that return to activity, particularly high-level sports, may be less predictable.

DISCLOSURE

The author has nothing to disclose.

REFERENCES

1. Dameron TB Jr. Fractures of the proximal fifth metatarsal: selecting the best treatment option. J Am Acad Orthop Surg 1995;3:110–4.

2. Clapper MF, O'Brien TJ, Lyons PM. Fractures of the fifth metatarsal: analysis of a fracture registry. Clin Orthop Relat Res 1995;315:238–41.
3. Smith JW, Arnoczky SP, Hersh A. The intraosseous blood supply of the fifth metatarsal: implications for proximal fracture healing. Foot Ankle 1992;13(3):143–52.
4. Jones R. Fracture of the base of the fifth metatarsal by indirect violence. Ann Surg 1902;35:697–700.
5. Chuckpaiwong B, Queen RM, Easley ME, et al. Distinguishing Jones and proximal diaphyseal fractures of the fifth metatarsal. Clin Orthop Relat Res 2008; 466(8):1966–70.
6. Den Hartog BD. Fracture of the proximal fifth metatarsal. J Am Acad Orthop Surg 2009;17(7):458–64.
7. Hunt KJ, Anderson RB. Treatment of Jones fracture nonunions and refractures in the elite athlete. Am J Sports Med 2011;39(9):1948–54.
8. O'Malley M, DeSandis B, Allen A, et al. Operative treatment of fifth metatarsal jones fractures (zone II and III) in the NBA. Foot Ankle Int 2016;37(5):488–500.
9. Nunley JA, Glasson RR. A new option for intramedullary fixation of Jones fractures: the Charlotte Carolina Jones Fracture System. Foot Ankle Int 2008; 29(12):1216–21.
10. Granata JD, Berlet GC, Philbin TM, et al. Failed surgical management of acute proximal fifth metatarsal (Jones) fractures. Foot Ankle Spec 2015;12:454–9.
11. Larson CM, Almekinders LC, Taft TN, et al. Intramedullary screw fixation of Jones fractures. Analysis of failure. Am J Sports Med 2002;30:55–60.
12. Raikin SM, Slenker N, Ratigan B. The association of a varus hindfoot and fracture of the fifth metatarsal metaphyseal-diaphyseal junction. Am J Sports Med 2008; 36(7):1367–72.

Turf Toe, Traumatic Hallux Valgus, and Hallux Rigidus -What Can I Do After an Metatarsophalangeal Fusion?

Anish R. Kadakia, MD[a],*, Mohammed T. Alshouli, MD[b],
Mauricio P. Barbosa, MD[c], Daniel Briggs, MD[d],
Muhammad Mutawakkil, MD[d]

KEYWORDS

- Turf toe • Traumatic hallux valgus • Internal brace • Hallux rigidus
- Metatarsophalangeal joint • Fusion

KEY POINTS

- Injury to the hallux should not be taken lightly as even moderate dysfunction can compromise the weightbearing and force transmission through the first metatarsophalangeal (MTP) joint.
- This compromise will negatively impact the ability of the athlete to return to preinjury level of play.
- Early restoration of hallux ligamentous stability has a high percentage chance of return to high-level sports.
- In cases of delayed diagnosis with subsequent arthritis, a first MTP fusion can restore stability and significantly improve function and should not be considered only for patients who are low demand.

INTRODUCTION

Trauma to the first metatarsophalangeal (MTP) joint can be a disabling injury to the athlete secondary to the loss of function of hallux stability. More than half of the body weight transmits through the first MTP joint during gait. Under these conditions, it is not surprising that trauma to the first ray frequently disrupts the sesamoid and first

[a] Department of Orthopedic Surgery, Center for Comprehensive Orthopaedic and Spine Care, Northwestern Memorial Hospital, Northwestern University, 259 East Erie, 13th Floor, Chicago, IL 60611, USA; [b] Prince Mohammed Bin AbdulAziz Hospital, Imam Bin Saud University, College of Medicine, Dar Aloloom University, College of Medicine, Riyadh, Saudi Arabia; [c] Orthobone Clinic, Asccociaiacao Beneficente Siria HCor, Sao Paul, Brazil; [d] Department of Orthopedic Surgery, Center for Comprehensive Orthopaedic and Spine Care, Northwestern Memorial Hospital, 259 East Erie, 13th Floor, Chicago, IL 60611, USA
* Corresponding author.
E-mail addresses: Kadak259@gmail.com; Akadaki1@nm.org

Clin Sports Med 39 (2020) 801–818
https://doi.org/10.1016/j.csm.2020.07.007
0278-5919/20/© 2020 Elsevier Inc. All rights reserved.
sportsmed.theclinics.com

MTP joint complex. Loss of stability to the hallux can have a significant negative impact on athletic ability and has been known to limit the ability to return to high-level sports for some athletes. Ligamentous instability from trauma to the hallux can result in primarily sagittal plane instability (turf toe) and the less commonly recognized coronal and sagittal instability (traumatic hallux valgus). Hallux rigidus results in pain and restriction of normal motion of the hallux that may not directly cause instability. However, it effectively limits the patient's ability to transmit force through the hallux. This results in decreased pushoff and transfer of force to the lateral border of the foot. Arthrodesis of the hallux is commonly viewed as an operation for sedentary patients that will severely limit activity; however, given the improvement in stability and minimization of pain, most patients are able to improve to their activity level significantly, understanding that normal cannot be achieved.

This article will focus on functional impact and surgical treatment options of hallux instability and arthritis in the athlete.

Turf Toe and Traumatic Hallux Valgus Background

In 1976, Bowers and Martin were the first to describe plantar capsular-ligamentous injury of the first MTP joint related to hard artificial surfaces and insubstantial footwear.[1] Turf toe is a general term used to describe various injuries to the hallux plantar capsule, plantar muscles, and the sesamoid complex of the hallux metatarsophalangeal joint. More specifically, turf toe injury refers to tearing of the plantar plate complex, the sesamoid-phalangeal ligament and capsule connecting the sesamoid to the base of the hallux proximal phalanx. Turf toe is a common sports injury that may lead to significant disability and loss of playing time and delayed recovery in professional athletes if not identified and treated promptly.[2] Review of published literature revealed no age or sex predilections for this injury. Mechanism of injury, playing surface, and individual biomechanics are reported predisposing factors to plantar plate injury, with a varying level of severity. These injuries are commonly described in American football players; 45% of professional football players surveyed reported suffering from turf toe.[3] Incidence increases with hard turf and flexible shoes. Athletes report difficulty in the push-off stage of running. However, this injury is also seen in other sports/activities such as basketball, soccer, and dance, but is much less frequent and is typically less severe. Coker and colleagues[2] reported a series of injuries in University of Arkansas football players. The authors described the severity of turf toe injury in terms of lost playing time and delayed return to play, even when compared with more common, but debilitating injuries.

The incidence of turf toe injuries among collegiate football players was initially believed to be 5 to 6 injuries per team per season; however, more recent studies estimate a lower incidence of turf toe injuries of 0.46 to 0.53 injuries per team per season. Harris and colleagues reported the overall reported incidence of turf toe injuries in American collegiate football players is 0.062 per 1000 athlete-exposures. Data analysis from the National Collegiate Athletic Association Injury Surveillance System also revealed that on average, 10.1 days were lost because of injury.[4,5]

Traumatic hallux valgus is often conceptualized as a variant of turf toe. Bowers and Martin first described turf toe in 1976.[1] They published a case series of 27 such injuries in West Virginia University football players occurring between 1970 and 1974. They described the mechanism as a forced dorsiflexion injury of the hallux MTP joint with the foot fixed and the heel elevated. Shortly thereafter, Coker and colleagues[2] described a distinct variant, a valgus injury at the MTP joint injuring the medial capsule, caused by sudden acceleration. They suggested such an injury presents with a more insidious onset than a pure hyperdorsiflexion injury. They advocated a first-line treatment of rest, splinting, and taping with a spring steel splint, and the consideration of surgical repair for athletes unable to jog at 3 weeks after injury. The authors' treatment regimen applied to all turf toe injuries and did not distinguish those with a traumatic valgus injury.

A series of 62 MTP joint injuries occurring in Rice University athletes from 1971 to 1985 included 2 athletes who developed late hallux valgus deformity 10 years after their MTP joint injuries.[5] The authors also noted several cases of early hallux rigidus and arthritic changes associated with turf toe, which they attributed to articular cartilage and subchondral bone injury. They posited that cartilage and subchondral bone injuries occur with complete capsuloligamentous disruption.

Turf toe injury can easily be overlooked, and therefore, requires a careful assessment of the initial presentation. Injury to the plantar ligamentous complex may result in primarily sagittal instability that is commonly thought of when considering the term turf toe. The authors will also discuss a described variant in detail that is commonly overlooked, traumatic hallux valgus, which results from a combined hyperdorsiflexion and eversion force to the great toe. This mechanism results in injury to the medial collateral ligament of the great toe in combination with the medial aspect of the plantar plate.

Anatomy

There are medial and lateral sesamoids named according to the anatomic location relative to the first metatarsal. Sesamoid ossification often occurs from multiple centers, and this may be the reason for the development of multipartite sesamoids. The 2 hallux sesamoids sit on the plantar surface directly underlying the first metatarsal head within a bony ridge known as the crista. The hallucal sesamoids articulate dorsally with the plantar surface of the distal aspect of the first metatarsal while the remainder of the respective sesamoid is enveloped within the medial and lateral tendons of the flexor hallucis brevis. The sesamoids are connected plantarly to each other centrally by the intersesamoid ligament, which acts as a pulley for the flexor hallucis longus tendon. Each sesamoid has an associated ligament inserting onto its respective side of the metatarsal head. The hallucal sesamoids are dynamically and statically stabilized by multiple ligaments and fibrous tissue connections to the MTP joint capsule and the plantar aponeurosis. The medial and lateral sesamoids have small attachments to the abductor and adductor hallucis tendons that insert on the medial and lateral bases of the proximal phalanx, respectively. These tendons, in addition to the collateral ligaments, provide stability in the axial plane for the first MTP. Distal to the sesamoids, the sesamoid-phalangeal ligament integrates with the collateral ligaments and tendons of the flexor hallucis brevis to form the plantar plate. Complete rupture of the plantar plate attachments may lead to a claw toe deformity with retraction of the sesamoids.[6–8] The complex network of ligamentous and tendinous attachments provide both static and dynamic mechanical stability to the hallux MTP joint.

Mechanism of Injury

Mechanism of injury, hard-playing surface, and individual biomechanics are reported predisposing factors to plantar plate injury. Rodeo and colleagues[3] reported that 85% of turf toe injuries result from hyperextension of the first MTP joint. Forty-five percent of professional football players surveyed reported suffering from turf toe. Less common mechanisms of injury include plantarflexion injury to the first MTP joint and varus or valgus stress injuries.[9] Hyperplantar-flexion injuries are more commonly seen in dancers and beach volleyball players.[10] This is widely believed to be related to the plantar plate rupture secondary to injury of the capsular-sesamoid-ligamentous complex. Clinically, in most shod athletic activities, the injury mechanism involves a pure hyperextension or combined extension with valgus stress and will be the focus of the further discussion.

History

There should be a high clinical suspicion for hallux MTP injuries in football players, soccer players, dancers, and those with high-demand activities that require foot impaction on a hard surface. Patients often report great toe pain after sustaining hyperdorsiflexion or forefoot valgus loading injury of the toe. The patient may complain of pain, swelling, and tenderness of the plantar aspect of the MTP, as well as an inability to push off with the great toe.[11]

Physical Examination

The patient should be evaluated for the presence of swelling and ecchymosis, or in severe cases, clawing or dislocation of the toe.[11] Joint structures should be palpated, including dorsal metatarsal head and neck, dorsal aspect of the proximal phalanx, the medial and lateral aspects of the MTP joint, and the plantar sesamoids to assess integrity and presence of tenderness to palpation.[11]

Stress tests should be performed to determine the stability of the hallux; however, this may be too painful at the time of injury. Delayed stress testing after a few days to allow for the acute pain to resolve or consideration for an examination under local anesthetic may provide a definitive examination for instability. A Lachman-type maneuver to assess the plantar plate with comparison to the contralateral noninjured extremity should be performed[11,12] (**Fig. 1**). Flexor hallucis brevis strength and integrity assessment is done by examining plantarflexion strength of the proximal phalanx against resistance.[11] An abduction stress test to assess the medial collateral ligament, medial capsule, and abductor hallucis is critical to determine if the injury is a traumatic hallux valgus variant. However, failure to demonstrate medial laxity on physical examination does not rule out ligamentous injury that may result in traumatic hallux valgus.[13] The examiner should also note any medial-sided ecchymoses to the MTP joint, as this may suggest injury to the MCL (**Table 1**).

Imaging

A routine 3-view (anterior to posterior, lateral, and oblique) conventional weight-bearing radiograph series of the foot can be used to assess the bony structures. Comparison radiographs of the contralateral foot are mandatory as patients with a rupture of the plantar plate will have proximal migration of one or both sesamoids.[14] A lateral stress test view at 45° of MTP joint hyperextension indirectly evaluates the functional integrity of the plantar plate – as a lack of distal migration of the sesamoids compared with the neutral lateral indicates complete rupture. Advanced imaging should be considered in suspected grade 2 or 3 injuries to fully determine the integrity of the plantar plate. MRI permits direct visualization of plantar plate tear,[15] concomitant related ligamentous and surrounding soft tissue injuries, and possible associated osseous or cartilaginous injury to the sesamoids or first metatarsal.[16] Specifically, MRI will help evaluate the presence of a complete rupture of the plantar plate versus an incomplete tear that will impact the treatment options for the patient. A computed tomography (CT) scan can be considered as well if there is any concern for bony injury to the dorsal metatarsal head or sesamoid integrity.

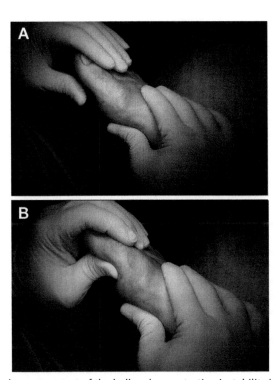

Fig. 1. Positive Lachman type test of the hallux demonstrating instability in the sagittal plan. This finding can be seen in turf toe and traumatic hallux valgus. Note the dorsal translation (*B*) compared with the nonstress examination (*A*).

Table 1
Turf toe injury classification by McCormick and Anderson

Grade of Injury	Description
Grade I -strain	Capsular ligamentous complex sprain: localized pain, minimum swelling, minimal ecchymosis; no articular instability/no detectable injuries on clinical examination and by imaging
Grade II – partial tear	Partial tear of the capsular ligamentous complex (partial articular instability): diffuse pain, moderate swelling, local ecchymosis; restricted motion because of pain; detectable ligamentous injuries on clinical examination and by imaging
Grade III – complete tear	Total rupture of capsular ligamentous complex: intense pain, evident swelling, ecchymosis; movement restricted by pain, positive vertical Lachman test (frank articular instability); possible associated lesions; lateral (varus) or medial (valgus) capsular ligamentous injury; sesamoid fracture or diastasis of a bipartite sesamoid; articular cartilage lesion or subchondral osseous edema

From McCormick JJ, and Anderson RB: Rehabilitation following turf toe injury and plantar plate repair. Clin Sports Med 2010; 29: pp. 313-323; with permission.

TREATMENT

No prospective, randomized trials exist that evaluate or compare treatment for turf toe injuries. However, small retrospective case series (Level IV evidence) universally support nonoperative management for grade I and II injuries. One case series supported operative treatment for grade III injuries.[17]

Bowers and colleagues,[1] Coker and colleagues,[2] Clanton and Ford,[18–20] and George and colleagues[4] have reported their experiences in treating patients with turf toe injuries These studies revealed that turf toe injury is more frequent in athletes, particularly football players, and the majority can be managed with nonoperative treatment with the ability to return to play in a few weeks after injury with toe splint and special shoes. However, most of these cases were grades 1 or 2 turf toe injuries with no reported radiological data about the severity of the injury to indicate the presence or absence of a completely torn plantar plate or capsular-ligamentous complex.

Coker and colleagues[2] reported that few cases underwent surgery, which was reserved for patients who complained of significant pain beyond 3 weeks of injury. However, the demographics of these patients and clinical indications of the operative treatment were not fully described in their study, and this makes it unclear when to proceed for surgery.

Clanton and Ford[18] have reported 1 case with an avulsion fracture of the first metatarsal that underwent operative treatment. They reported return to play after 56 days, and noted that 10 of 20 patients who sustained a turf toe injury had continued pain and symptoms at 5 years follow-up.

A review of recent literature showed that few studies (Level IV evidence) have reported results of operative treatment of turf toe with successful outcomes and the ability to return to sports.

Anderson[21] reported a case series of 9 patients who underwent surgery for grade III injuries with radiographic evidence of sesamoid migration and disruption of the plantar soft tissue complex on MRI scans. The duration from injury to surgery ranged from 1 week to 7 months, with follow-up from 1 to 10 years. The repair of the plantar plate complex was performed in all patients. In 4 patients (44%), sesamoidectomies were also performed because of fragmentation or degeneration, with abductor hallucis tendon transferred to fill in the defect in 3 of these patients. Seven patients (78%) were able to return to a full level of activity with minimal pain. The remaining 2 patients were unable to return to full athletic activity, one because of persistent pain despite a stable toe, whereas the other developed severe hallux rigidus.

Traumatic hallux valgus appears to have a less favorable outcome with nonoperative treatment when compared with a pure hyperdorsiflexion injury.[21] In his series, Anderson recommended acute surgical intervention for patients with traumatic hallux valgus with a slight modification of the repair required for grade III turf toe injuries (Level IV evidence).[21] Douglas and colleagues[22] reported restoration of stability and normal range of motion after surgical repair of the medial collateral ligament 4 weeks after injury in a soccer player with medial collateral ligament disruption on MRI (Level V evidence). Fabeck and colleagues[23] reported a single case of delayed reconstruction with a modified McBride 6 months after a valgus injury to the great toe (Level V evidence).

AUTHOR'S PREFERRED METHOD
Conservative Treatment

In cases of grade I injuries, along with the initial supportive measures (eg, rest, ice, compression and elevation), the great toe usually gets benefit from immobilization using a walking boot, short leg cast for pain, and swelling management for 24 to 48 hours. This can be changed to toe taping in a slightly plantarflexed position and return to play with taping or a custom orthotic to limit dorsiflexion if pain-free with weightbearing and range of motion. Depending on severity, most patients are able to return to protected play within 2 to 3 weeks as symptoms resolve.

For all patients who have a suspected grade 2 injury, the authors prefer to obtain an MRI to further delineate the injury to the soft tissue. If there is no evidence of injury to the medial collateral ligament (traumatic hallux valgus), incomplete tear of the plantar plate, and no bony injury, the authors initiate a nonsurgical protocol. They divide the recovery into 3 phases as has been previously described.[18]

The goal of phase 1 is protection and swelling and pain management, which can be achieved using a walking boot, short leg cast, or a toe spica extension in slight flexion/valgus, to keep the plantar soft tissues in a rested position; this usually lasts up to 3 days.[18]

The goal of phase 2 is to restore pain-free functional range of motion and ability to walk without pain. Active toe flexion should be initiated as soon as swelling permits, and active and passive dorsiflexion should be limited until adequate plantar healing has occurred. These restrictions are used in conjunction with toe taping and the use of rigid, stiff-soled shoes to limit excessive first MTP dorsiflexion during weightbearing activities; this may last up to 4 weeks.

In phase 3, when the patient demonstrates a pain-free range of motion on clinical testing and low-impact activities, he or she should be prepared to return to sport. There is a general consensus that 60° of painless dorsiflexion along with painless weightbearing is the appropriate criteria for return to play. Although this is not based on a body of scientific evidence, the authors do follow this algorithm in cases of grade 2 injuries. All players are protected with a combination of taping and forefoot support with a custom orthotic that limits dorsiflexion of the hallux.

The role for nonoperative treatment of acute traumatic hallux valgus or progressive post-traumatic hallux valgus is negligible. In the case of medial-sided hallux MTP injury significant enough to cause deformity, it is unlikely that nonoperative treatment will be adequate for anatomic healing. Although the detailed natural history of traumatic hallux valgus is not described in the literature, it is thought that left untreated, the injury will likely go on to post-traumatic arthritis with limited options for joint preservation.

Surgical Treatment

The combination of the limited literature and the authors' own personal experience has led them to encourage surgical treatment for all grade 3 and cases of traumatic hallux valgus. The authors have noted that conservative treatment leads to persistent inability to play at the patient's desired level, and delayed reconstruction is more difficult with a less predictable outcome compared with acute management. The resultant loss of hallux stability and plantarflexion strength, as well as traumatic hallux valgus or claw toe deformity, may result in the inability to return to competitive play in high-level athletes. Hence, the surgical treatment discussed will focus on acute treatment of a turf toe injury and chronic reconstruction of delayed traumatic hallux valgus.

Acute turf toe repair

Surgical treatment of a turf toe is the most reproducible method to return an athlete to high-level play despite the risks that are involved. Two primary incisions have been discussed, a J-type incision that has a medial linear incision, along the medial sesamoid that is taken transversely distally along the plantar flexion crease directed toward

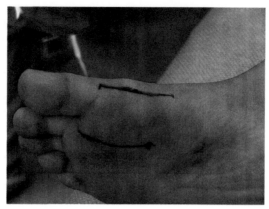

Fig. 2. Dual incisions allow for excellent exposure with a decreased risk of iatrogenic injury to the lateral plantar digital nerve.

the first web space. Although this incision does allow for excellent exposure, a large subcutaneous flap is required to expose the fibular sesamoid. Additionally, the transverse nature of the incision places the lateral plantar digital nerve at risk of injury. Therefore, the authors prefer a dual-incision approach that has been described to expose both the tibial and fibular sesamoid/plantar plate complex (**Fig. 2**). Given the location of the incision, the authors prefer a supine approach with mild external rotation of the affected limb to allow better exposure of the medial MTP approach. Although a prone approach can be considered, the authors have not found this to be necessary and have concerns regarding access to the dorsal MTP joint for treatment of osteochondral defects or osteophytes. Sharp dissection is taken through the skin, followed by the use of blunt dissection until the medial digital nerve is identified (**Fig. 3**). Laterally, the nerve may not be directly visualized depending on the location of the incision. The authors prefer a slightly more laterally based incision just lateral to the most prominent part of the fat pad. This places the incision lateral to

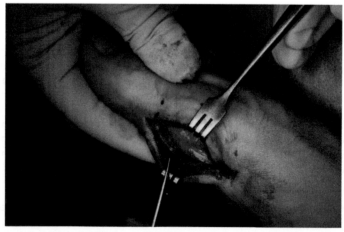

Fig. 3. Medial approach requires identification of the medial plantar digital nerve (freer elevator) that should be retracted inferiorly.

the lateral plantar digital nerve. A detailed understanding of the location of the nerve relative to the sesamoid will minimize the risk of injury (**Fig. 4**). In the setting of an acute injury, the disruption of the plantar plate complex is evident with the presence of hematoma and a clear defect in the capsuloligamentous complex. The rupture of the ligament may occur in 3 different locations if the sesamoid has not been fractured: distal avulsion from the phalanx, intrasubstance, or proximally from the sesamoid. For disruption from the phalanx, the use of a suture anchor for repair will suffice. The authors prefer a small suture anchor given the small bony footprint. Intrasubstance ruptures are more easily repaired directly with the use of size 0 absorbable or nonabsorbable suture. Given the small area that is available for visualization, the use of a 5/8 curved needle facilitates the ability to grasp both ends of the tissue with the needle's tight radius of curvature. Proximal avulsion is treated with either a small drill hole or small suture anchor. The authors prefer the use of small drill hole in the sesamoid to pass a suture (**Fig. 5**). In most cases, the medial soft tissue is more amenable to repair given the ease of visualization. Following completion of the direct repair, the remaining soft tissue should be reinforced to complete the repair and improve the mechanical rigidity of the construct (**Fig. 6**).

A complicating factor that can occur with turf toe is fracture of the sesamoid, given the difficulty of ORIF of the bone, owing to its small size and frequent comminution in these injuries. For small pole fracture where more than 75% of the bone is intact, removal of the smaller fragment and repair are effective. Excision of the damaged sesamoid is required in the setting of comminution with imbrication of the remaining soft tissue. Excision of 1 sesamoid and imbrication of the remaining soft tissue are effective as ORIF of the sesamoid is not predictable (**Fig. 7**). Rarely, there is significant comminution of both sesamoids that prevents salvage of either sesamoid. The primary concern is that a medial and lateral soft tissue repair with concomitant removal of the sesamoids will not result in sufficient mechanical stability to the joint. To augment the soft tissue repair medially, as laterally it is more difficult given the limited window of visualization, transfer of the abductor into the soft tissue defect has been described.[24] Although this technique may provide for stability in these difficult situations, this method is nonanatomic and can result in weakness of soft tissue fixation. The advent

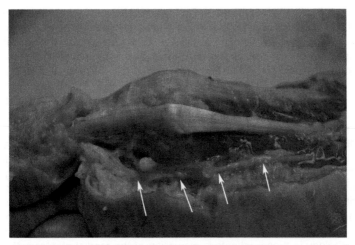

Fig. 4. Anatomic specimen identifying the lateral plantar digital nerve (*arrows*). Note the location immediately lateral to the fibular sesamoid.

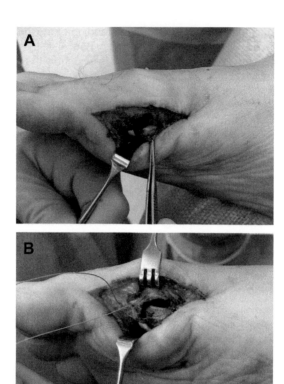

Fig. 5. Proximal pole avulsion of the plantar plate with visualization of the flexor hallucis longus (A). The use of a transverse drill hole for suture placement allows for a stable and reproducible method of reconstruction in this setting (B).

of the Internal Brace (Arthrex, Naples, Florida) has allowed for improved mechanical stability of soft tissue reconstruction, most commonly used for lateral ankle instability. The authors have used this implant to provide improved mechanical stability for the medial capsular repair in the setting of hallux valgus with excellent success. Taking the same concept to these difficult situations, the authors have developed a technique to use the internal brace to supplement the soft tissue repair for turf toe by placing the implant in a more plantar and medial position. Use of this technique may mitigate the need to transfer the abductor, or if a transfer is chosen, will provide superior mechanical strength to the repair.

The authors have primarily used this augmentation technique for the treatment of traumatic hallux valgus. As stated previously, in most cases of traumatic hallux valgus, given that the patient is able to bear weight after the injury, most presentations appear once the condition has reached the chronic stage with deformity. Prior surgical consideration was to treat this as a standard hallux valgus with a distal osteotomy and soft tissue release. However, distal metatarsal osteotomy is not without risks and may lead to stiffness of the great toe and in rare cases avascular necrosis. The primary pathology in these patients is disruption of the medial plantar soft tissue restraints that are adequately treated neither with a simple imbrication of the tissue

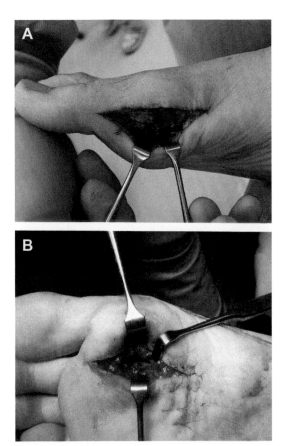

Fig. 6. Final appearance of the medial repair (*A*) and lateral repair (*B*) of a grade 3 turf toe that required excision of the fibular sesamoid.

nor the osteotomy. Therefore, in order to restore sagittal stability and correct coronal instability, augmented reconstruction of the soft tissue can be considered. A medial-based incision as would be used for a standard approach to the hallux is utilized. The authors prefer this incision over a more plantar-based incision to minimize injury the medial plantar nerve. The medial soft tissue is intact in a chronic situation with no clear defect present to imbricate. A plantar-based wedge of the medial capsule and plantar plate is excised to restore the stability of the hallux. The length of the plantar transverse limb is approximately 3 mm and can be increased if it is felt more imbrication is required. Multiple number 0 vicryl sutures are utilized in figure of 8 fashion to appose the tissue. Following completion of the suture repair, the hallux should rest in a slightly plantarflexed and adducted position (**Fig. 8**). The augmentation technique is then utilized to provide the mechanical support to allow for early range of motion and minimize the risk of correction loss secondary to loss of tissue apposition. The 3.5 mm interference screw is placed within the phalanx plantar medially (**Fig. 9**). The Fibertape (Arthrex) is then taken through the plantar tissue to ensure that the suture remains along the plantar medial aspect of the hallux and does not migrate dorsally. The proximal fixation is performed with another 3.5 mm interference screw within the metatarsal head. If fixation is insufficient, a 4.75 mm interference screw can be used

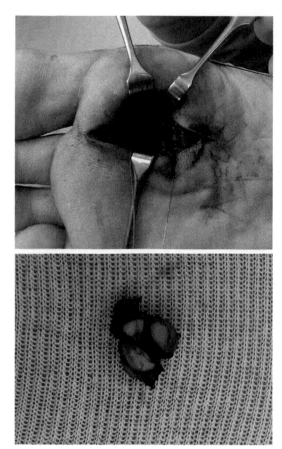

Fig. 7. Sesamoid fractures in the setting of a grade III turf toe are best treated with excision and imbrication of the remaining flexor hallucis brevis to close the large soft tissue defect.

proximally without any difficulty (**Fig. 10**). Care must be taken not to place the interference screw proximal to the metatarsal head, as the diaphysis is hollow, and the fixation from these devices is not ideal in this location. Although it can be used in the diaphysis if necessary, it is critical in this case not to overpenetrate the medial cortex, as loss of fixation may occur. Tensioning the construct is a critical aspect in all soft tissue reconstructions to ensure effectiveness of the augmentation. Care should be taken not to allow overtension of the tape during proximal fixation. Travel of the tape into the hole may result in a significant varus position of the hallux. Preliminary tensioning should be performed with the tape held along the length of the insertion device, marking the location of the laser line on the tape with a marking pen. The tip of the insertion device is taken to the level of the mark, and the interference screw is then inserted in standard fashion. However, this technique is not foolproof, and many surgeons prefer to place the tip just shy of the mark to minimize the risk of laxity. Therefore, the authors prefer to have an assistant stabilize the hallux or use a transarticular 0.062 smooth K-wire during proximal fixation. Although a transarticular K-wire may cause trauma to the cartilage, the authors have not found this to be a clinical issue. The benefit/risk of using a K-wire must be weighed against over- or undertensioning of the repair.

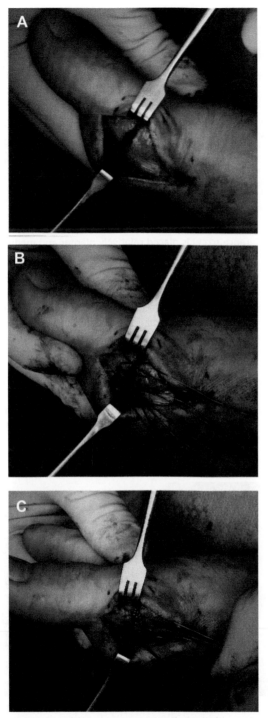

Fig. 8. Chronic traumatic hallux valgus exposure will demonstrate an intact, however patulous medial collateral ligament and plantar plate. A plantar based wedge of medial capsule is excised in order to restore the capsule to a more function length (*A*). Following excision, multiple figure of 8 sutures are used to imbricate the tissue (*B*). Note the new neutral resting position of the hallux following tightening of the sutures (*C*).

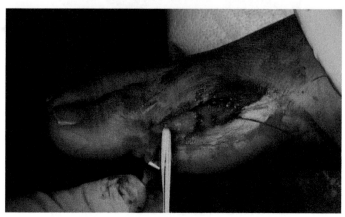

Fig. 9. The 3.5 interference screw is placed relatively plantar and medial into the proximal phalanx.

Postoperatively, a flat surgical shoe or heel wedge weightbearing shoe is utilized. Although a flat postoperative shoe will not damage the repair, given the plantar incision, the postoperative pain is minimized with a heel wedge device. In cases of both turf toe and traumatic hallux valgus, the authors also utilize a toe spacer between the hallux and second toe. Transition to a flat postoperative shoe may be used as comfort dictates following week 2. The use of a gym shoe with a carbon fiber plate is considered at week 6 and initiating of physical therapy for nonimpact activity, with a focus on balance and weightbearing through the hallux. For the subset of patients with traumatic hallux valgus, the silicone toe spacer is used until 3 months postoperatively. After 3 months postoperatively, unrestricted activity as tolerated is allowed; however, the use of a carbon fiber plate is encouraged for a total of 6 months.

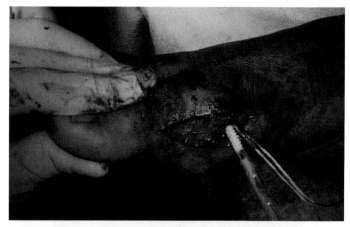

Fig. 10. Following imbrication of the medial capsule and plantar plate, the suture tape device should be tensioned with the hallux in a neutral position. Overcorrection of the hallux should be avoided, as the goal of the augmentation is to act as a check rein to the primary soft tissue reconstruction. A 0.045 K wire is placed across the joint temporarily if required during placement to minimize the risk of overtensioning.

CLINICAL RESULTS

Nery and colleagues have reported a case series of 24 patients who were treated with MTP1 joint instability. All patients were performing sports activities when they were injured. Injuries were classified as grade I (2 patients—8%), grade II (8 patients—33%), and grade III (14 patients—59%) lesions. All patients with grades I and II were treated conservatively, whereas those classified as grade III were treated surgically. Significant improvement in AOFAS hallux scores reported after treatment were 51 to 84 (P<.001) and 36 to 81 (P<.001) for conservative and surgical groups, respectively. However, 4 patients with grade 3 injuries (29%) and 2 patients with grade 2 injuries (20%) did not resume their previous activities. They concluded that both forms of treatment could lead to satisfactory results if well conducted. The correct identification, classification, and grading of first MTP instability help in decision making and selection of adequate treatment.[25]

Hainsworth and McKinley[26] published a systematic review aimed at addressing in what circumstances operative intervention is indeed superior to conservative management of turf toe in adults. The primary outcome measure was the time to return to preinjury activity, and the secondary outcome was the time to symptom resolution. They reported 7 studies met the inclusion criteria. Three patients were successfully managed conservatively, returning to athletic activity, on average, at 12 weeks. Seventeen patients underwent surgical intervention with an average return to athletic activity at 18 weeks. They concluded that operative intervention was shown to give a successful outcome in patients with grade 3 turf toe injuries or those who failed conservative management. However, there is insufficient evidence to determine whether operative intervention is superior to conservative management.

Smith and Waldrop have reported a cohort study of 15 patients operatively treated for grade 3 turf toe injuries. Results demonstrate good clinical outcomes were achieved with an operative repair of grade 3 injuries with average AOFAS hallux score of 91.3, VAS score of 0.8 with activity, and the average missed playing time of 16.5 weeks.[27]

Douglas and colleagues[22] published a case report of an acute medial collateral ligament (MCL) disruption in an elite soccer player that occurred after he was slide tackled during practice. The patient presented 4 days following the injury with pain and swelling at the medial MTP joint but with no instability on examination. The patient continued to complain of pain and subjective instability for the next month. Repeat clinical examinations were negative for instability, but MRI demonstrated a tear of the MCL on T1-weighted and short tau inversion recovery sequences. The authors repaired the MCL with 0-Ethibond suture, and at 6 weeks the patient had no subjective complaints.

Covell and colleagues[28] reported a case series of 19 elite athletes treated for traumatic hallux valgus. The series included 12 National Football League athletes, 6 college athletes, and 1 high school athlete, who were all treated by a single surgeon between 2006 and 2015. Of the athletes who could recall the specific date of their injury, the average time to surgery was 4.5 months. The surgical repair consisted of medial eminence resection of the first metatarsal head, medial ligamentous and capsular reefing, flexor halluces brevis repair, and a modified McBride. Fourteen of the 19 patients returned to their preinjury level of sport, at an average of 3.4 months from the time of surgery.

Function After First Metatarsophalangeal Fusion

The concept of doing a fusion of the great toe is seen as an end to athletic activities of the patient, conjuring up images of cosmetically unappealing shoes and sedentary activity. Fortunately, these presumptions about function following a first MTP arthrodesis are not accurate, and a significant preservation of hallux function occurs with this procedure.

Da Cunha and colleagues[29] reported about returning to sports after first MTP fusion in young patients and showed that no physical activities were affected after the surgery, and they were able to do 21 different activities after fusion. The more common sports pre and postoperatively were walking, biking, swimming, weightlifting, running and golf. Even patients engaged in high-impact sports like soccer, running, football, basketball, and dancing did not have problems with return. Patients were able to return to about 86% of the reported physical activities within 12 months after surgery. Fifty-six percent of these patients had high and very high level of activities postoperatively from 5 to more than 10 hours per week. A striking 96% of the patients were satisfied with the result of the surgery in regards to return to sports and physical activities.

Brodsky and colleagues[30] observed improvement in propulsive power and stability during gait analysis of 23 patients with first MTP joint fusion. This study demonstrated that ankle push-off power and single limb support increased after first MTP fusion. In another study in 2005, Brodsky noticed improvement in functional outcome and pain relief after first MTP fusion, with most patients able to return to sports such as tennis, golfing, hiking, and jogging.[31]

Ellington and colleagues[32] also reported their outcomes for first MTP fusion in 98 patients treated for hallux valgus, hallux rigidus, revisions, and neuromuscular etiology. They employed a different fixation technique with dorsal plating. They reported improvement in AOFAS, VAS pain scores, shoe wear, and physical activity. Eighty-nine percent of patients reported good to excellent results.

In contrast, Daniilidis and colleagues[33] reported a prospective study with 23 patients who underwent first MTP joint arthroplasty and showed good clinical and functional results after 18 months. However, the study demonstrated a decrease in return to recreational sports activities in relation to the preoperative state.

For patients with advanced stage hallux rigidus who want to do some sports after the surgery, even with high impact, there is an abundance of evidence to support that arthrodesis is the best and safest option of treatment. Lleyton Hewitt is an Australian professional tennis player and a former World Number 1 who was advised to avoid first MTP fusion, because it could potentially be career ending. He eventually underwent hallux arthrodesis for his left foot in 2012 for unrelenting pain that was no longer responsive to pain killers and injections. After a rigorous rehabilitation, he was able to return to the sport and record his first win just 3.5 months after surgery. He went on to win subsequent Wimbledon matches that year and continued to play professional tennis until his retirement in 2016.[34,35]

SUMMARY

Turf toe injuries should be recognized and treated early to prevent long-term disability. Clinical presentation, the mechanism of injury, and appropriate imaging help in the timely diagnosis. The accurate clinical assessment and early radiological evaluation of appropriate cases are important steps in differentiating the different grades of turf toe injuries. Both conservative and surgical treatments play major role in getting athletes back to their preinjury level if directed to the right group of injury at the right time. There are more recent reported case series and systemic reviews that encourage operative treatment as early as possible for grade III turf toe injury. This would help minimize the loss of playtime and earlier return to preinjury level. More studies should evaluate the rehabilitation protocols after conservative and operative treatments for better functional outcomes. If the patient presents late from a traumatic hallux injury with subsequent degenerative changes or has hallux rigidus from other etiologies, a first MTP arthrodesis should be considered to minimize pain and improve function. Although not all patients will return to high-level activity, an arthrodesis does not imply that athletic activity must be ceased.

DISCLOSURE

Arthrex, consultant, speaker's bureau; Depuy, royalties; Acumed, - royalties.

REFERENCES

1. Bowers KD, Martin RB. Turf-toe: a shoe-surface related football injury. Med Sci Sports 1976;8:81–3.
2. Coker TP, Arnold JA, Weber DL. Traumatic lesions of the metatarsophalangeal joint of the great toe in athletes. Am J Sports Med 1978;6:326–34.
3. Rodeo SA, O'Brien S, Warren RF, et al. Turf-toe: an analysis of metatarsophalangeal joint sprains in professional football players. Am J Sports Med 1990;18:280–5.
4. George E, Harris HS, Dragoo JL, et al. Incidence and risk factors for turf toe injuries in intercollegiate football: data from the National Collegiate Athletic Association Injury Surveillance System. Foot Ankle Int 2013;35:108–15.
5. Clanton TO, Butler JE, Eggert A. Injuries to the metatarsophalangeal joints in athletes. Foot Ankle 1986;7(3):162-176.
6. Kadakia AR. Disorders of the hallucal sesamoids, presentation, imaging and treatment of common musculoskeletal conditions, Chapter 112. 2012. p. 669–74.
7. Bock P, Kristen K, Kroner A, et al. Hallux valgus and cartilage degeneration in the first metatarsophalangeal joint. J Bone Surg Br 2004;86B:669–73.
8. Coughlin M. Athletic injury to the first metatarsal phalangeal joint. Med Chir Pied 2005;21:65–72.
9. Allen LR, Flemming D, Sanders TG. Turf toe: Ligamentous injury of the first metatarsophalangeal joint. Mil Med 2004;69:19–25.
10. Watson TS, Anderson RB, Davis WH. Periarticular injuries to the hallux metatarsophalangeal joint in athletes. Foot Ankle Clin 2000;5:687–713.
11. VanPelt MD, Saxena A, Allen MA. Turf toe injuries. In: Saxena A,, editor. Sports medicine and arthroscopic surgery of the foot and ankle. London: Springer-Verlag; 2013. p. 13–27.
12. Frimenko RE, Lievers W, Coughlin MJ, et al. Etiology and biomechanics of first metatarsophalangeal joint sprains (turf toe) in athletes. Crit Rev Biomed Eng 2012;40:43–61.
13. Robinson D, Heller E, Garti A. Sesamoid complex disruption as a cause of hallux valgus: report of three cases. Foot (Edinb) 2012;22(4):322–5.
14. McCormick JJ, Anderson RB. Rehabilitation following turf toe injury and plantar plate repair. Clin Sports Med 2010;29:313–23.
15. Tewes DPD, Fischer DAD, Fritts HMH, et al. MRI findings of acute turf toe. A case report and review of anatomy. Clin Orthop Relat Res 1994;304:200–3.
16. Crain JM, Phancao JP, Stidham K. MR Imaging of turf toe. Magn Reson Imaging Clin N Am 2008;16:93–103.
17. Kadakia AR, Molloy A. Current concepts review: traumatic disorders of the first metatarsophalangeal joint and sesamoid complex. Foot Ankle Int 2011;32:834–9.
18. Clanton TOT, Ford JJJ. Turf toe injury. Clin Sports Med 1994;13:731–41.

19. McCormick JJ, Anderson RB. The great toe: failed turf toe, chronic turf toe, and complicated sesamoid injuries. Foot Ankle Clin 2009;14:135–50.

20. Maglaya CL, Cook C, Zarzour H, et al. Return to division 1A football following a metatarsophalangeal joint dorsal dislocation. N Am J Sports Phys Ther 2010;5: 131–42.

21. Anderson RB. Turf toe injuries of the hallux metatarsophalangeal joint. Tech Foot Ankle Surg 2002;1:102–11.

22. Douglas DP, Davidson DM, Robinson JE, et al. Rupture of the medial collateral ligament of the first MTP joint in a professional soccer player. J Foot Ankle Surg 1997;36(5):388–90.

23. Fabeck LG, Zekhini C, Farrokh D. Traumatic hallux valgus following rupture of the medial collateral ligament of the first metatarsophalangeal joint: a case report. J Foot Ankle Surg 2002;41(2):125–8.

24. McCormick JJ, Anderson RB. Turf toe: anatomy, diagnosis, and treatment. Sports Health 2010;2(6):487-494.

25. Nery C, Fonseca LF, Gonçalves JP, et al. First MTP joint instability — expanding the concept of "turf-toe" injuries. Foot Ankle Surg 2020;26(1):47–53.

26. Hainsworth L, McKinley J. The management of turf toe – a systematic review. Br J Sports Med 2017;B51:A7.3–8.

27. Smith K, Waldrop N. Operative outcomes of grade 3 turf toe injuries in competitive football players. Foot Ankle Int 2018;39(9):1076-1081.

28. Covell DJ, Lareau CR, Anderson RB. Operative treatment of traumatic hallux valgus in elite athletes. Foot Ankle Int 2017;38(6):590–5.

29. Da Cunha RJ, Macmahon A, Jones MT, et al. Return to sports and physical activities after first metatarsophalangeal joint arthrodesis in young patients. Foot Ankle Int 2019;40(7):745–52.

30. Brodsky JW, Baum BS, Pollo FE, et al. Prospective gait analysis in patients with first metatarsophalangeal joint arthrodesis for hallux rigidus. Foot Ankle Int 2007;28(2):162–5.

31. Brodsky JW, Passmore RN, Pollo FE, et al. Functional outcome of arthrodesis of the first metatarsophalangeal joint using parallel screw fixation. Foot Ankle Int 2005;26(2):140–6.

32. Ellington JK, Jones CP, Cohen BE, et al. Review of 107 hallux MTP joint arthrodesis using dome-shaped reamers and a stainless-steel dorsal plate. Foot Ankle Int 2010;31(5):385-390.

33. Daniilidis K, Martinelli N, Denaro V, et al. Recreational sport activity after total replacement of the first metatarsophalangeal joint: a prospective study. Int Orthopaedics 2010;34(7):973–9.

34. Available at: https://www.abc.net.au/news/2013-06-25/hewitt-defies-seven-surgeons-of-doom/4778202#:%7E:text=Seven%20surgeons%20told%20Lleyton%20Hewitt,be%20reckoned%20with%20once%20again.%26text=%22There%20were%20two%20surgeons%2C%20the,it%20and%20one%20other%20guy.

35. Cody EA, Do HT, Koltsov JCB, et al. Influence of Diagnosis and Other Factors on Patients' Expectations of Foot and Ankle Surgery. Foot Ankle Int 2018;39(6): 641-648.

Posterior Tibial Tendon Transfer for Common Peroneal Nerve Injury

Joseph S. Park, MD[a],*, Michael J. Casale, MD[b]

KEYWORDS

- Posterior tibial tendon • Foot drop • Knee dislocation • Common peroneal nerve

KEY POINTS

- The incidence of common peroneal nerve dysfunction after knee dislocation or multiligament knee injury ranges from 4% to 40%.
- The mainstay of nonoperative treatment is an ankle–foot orthosis and close observation for interval improvement in symptoms.
- In patients with continued functional deficits who fail nonoperative treatment, posterior tibial tendon transfer to the dorsum of the foot is an excellent option.
- These authors favor passing the tendon through the interosseous membrane and into the lateral cuneiform as described in this article.
- Short- and long-term studies have shown substantial improvements in functional outcomes as well as functional restoration of ankle dorsiflexion strength and range of motion.

 Video content accompanies this article at http://www.sportsmed.theclinics.com.

INTRODUCTION

Once thought to be rare injuries, knee dislocations and multiligament knee injuries are now believed to account for up to 0.2% of traumatic orthopedic injuries.[1,2] The incidence of common peroneal nerve (CPN) dysfunction after knee dislocation varies widely in the literature from 4% to 40% and encompasses a range of severity from spontaneously resolving neurapraxia to permanent, complete injury.[3] Arom and colleagues[4] describes knee dislocation as a "spectrum of injuries, rather than a discrete entity," depending on several different factors, including direction of dislocation,

[a] Foot and Ankle Division, Department of Orthopedic Surgery, University of Virginia Health System, 400 Ray C. Hunt Drive, Suite 330, Charlottesville, VA 22908, USA; [b] Raleigh Orthopedic Clinic, Foot and Ankle Surgery, 3001 Edwards Mill Road, Raleigh, NC 27612, USA
* Corresponding author.
E-mail address: jsp3x@virginia.edu

Clin Sports Med 39 (2020) 819–828
https://doi.org/10.1016/j.csm.2020.07.003
0278-5919/20/© 2020 Elsevier Inc. All rights reserved.

disruption of cruciate or collateral ligaments, and associated nerve or vascular injury. The most commonly used classification system was proposed by Schenck[5] and is shown in **Table 1**.

Moatshe and colleagues[6] showed an overall rate of peroneal nerve injury in knee dislocation of 19.2%, with 10.9% being partial deficits and 8.3% being complete deficits. Additionally, they showed a 42 times greater likelihood of having a peroneal nerve injury in patients with a KD-IIIL (bicruciate disruption with posterolateral corner injury) pattern.

Keating provided a classification system based on the mechanism of injury and energy involved[7]:

1. High energy: usually motor vehicle collisions, accounting for approximately 50% of injuries
2. Low energy: usually sports injuries, accounting for approximately 33% of injuries
3. Ultra-low energy: usually ground level falls, accounting for approximately 12% of injuries

Furthermore, Stewart and colleagues[8] showed that neurologic injury in knee dislocation occurs more commonly with low-energy (7%) and ultra-low energy mechanisms (6%) compared with high-energy mechanisms (3%). For the ultra-low energy group, obesity was found to be a risk factor for neurologic as well as vascular injury.

The CPN is most commonly injured because of the anatomic constraints on its ability to accommodate traumatic changes in knee position proximally at the fibular neck and distally at the intermuscular septum. Historically, the prognosis for patients with CPN dysfunction and foot drop after multiligament knee injury has been poor; studies have shown worse results with regard to function, pain, and overall quality of life compared with patients without neurologic injury.[3] When comparing partial versus complete nerve palsy groups, Krych and colleagues[9] showed a significantly increased rate of recovery of active dorsiflexion in partial CPN injury patients. The authors could not find a significant difference in knee outcome scores (International Knee Documentation Committee or Lysholm scores) for CPN injury patients compared with those without nerve injury.

Although ankle–foot orthoses have traditionally been used to treat foot drop, multiple studies have shown that posterior tibial tendon transfer to the dorsum of the foot can provide encouraging functional outcomes. A 2016 study by Werner and colleagues[3] showed improved ankle dorsiflexion and sagittal plane kinematics, and decreased compensatory hip and knee flexion in patients who underwent posterior tibial tendon transfer compared with patients treated nonoperatively with orthoses.

Table 1	
Schenck classification for knee dislocations	
Type	**Description**
KD I	Knee dislocation with either cruciate intact
KD II	Bicruciate injury with collaterals intact
KD III	Bicruciate Injury with one collateral ligament injury KD IIIM – bicruciate injury with medial collateral injury KD IIIL – bicruciate injury with lateral collateral ligament injury
KD IV	Bicruciate injury with both medial/lateral collateral ligament injury
KD V	Periarticular fracture dislocation

Associated injuries: C = arterial injury; N = neural injury.

Additionally, Cho and colleagues[10] showed that posterior tibial tendon transfer resulted in consistent improvement in functional outcome scores, although transfer restored only 33% of dorsiflexion strength compared with the contralateral extremity.

There are many variations in the operative techniques for posterior tibial tendon transfer described in the literature. A 2018 cadaveric study by Wagner and colleagues[11] evaluated the biomechanical implications of different routes for the posterior tibial tendon, including circumtibial and transmembranous; they found the transmembranous route to be superior with regard to gliding resistance and final range of motion. Coughlin and associates[12] note that adequate passive dorsiflexion is essential to success, and posterior contracture release (via either a Strayer procedure or tendo-Achilles lengthening) must be performed to ensure active dorsiflexion.

EVALUATION AND MANAGEMENT

Frequently, patients with post-traumatic foot drop are referred to our practice for consideration for posterior tibial tendon transfer by the treating sports medicine surgeon. Direct communication with the referring surgeon should take place to better understand the intraoperative findings, especially the condition of the CPN at the time of knee reconstruction. At our institution, if a CPN injury is suspected, exploration and neurolysis of the CPN is routinely performed during the reconstructive knee procedure. If the nerve architecture is felt to be relatively well-preserved without extensive ecchymosis or notable stretch injury, nonoperative measures are used for 12 months before consideration of tendon transfer. **Fig. 1** demonstrates well-maintained

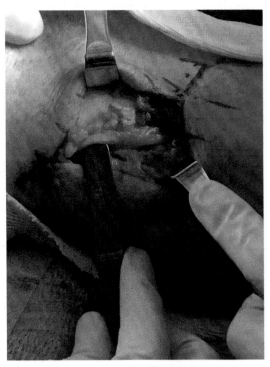

Fig. 1. Exploration of the CPN. Intact nerve visualized as it courses around the fibular neck, proximal (*left*) to distal (*right*).

architecture of the CPN during surgical exploration. In isolated cases of severe nerve injury or complete transection or discontinuity (**Figs. 2** and **3**), earlier surgical treatment with tendon transfer may be considered.

During the initial evaluation of the patient with multiligamentous knee injury and concomitant CPN injury, a thorough neurovascular examination must be performed and documented. Specifically, pulses, distal perfusion, capillary refill, and sensory/motor function must be evaluated. If there is concern for vascular compromise, urgent noninvasive vascular studies should be ordered, with vascular surgery consulted as necessary. Loss of active ankle, hallux, and lesser toe dorsiflexion, as well as loss of active hind-foot eversion, will be present with complete CPN injury. Sensory deficits are typically found for the deep peroneal and superficial peroneal nerve distributions, in addition to variable involvement of the sural nerve dermatome. This presents as absent or diminished sensation to the entire dorsum of the foot, including the first webspace, as well as the anterolateral distal one-third of the lower leg. It is important to document strength of the posterior tibial tendon (inversion/plantarflexion) as well as the hallux and lesser toe flexors. The posterior tibial tendon, flexor hallucis longus, and flexor digitorum longus are innervated by the tibial nerve, which is seldom injured in multiligament knee injuries. The absence of plantar sensation or inversion/flexion may suggest more proximal nerve injury related to lumbar spine or sciatic nerve injury or dysfunction.

If the posterior tibial tendon does not have full strength and cannot be instantly activated by the patient, physical therapy should be used to improve passive ankle dorsiflexion as well as to facilitate activation and strengthening of the posterior tibial tendon. Passive ankle dorsiflexion should be examined, with the knee in both extended and flexed positions. Isolated gastrocnemius contracture (ankle dorsiflexion limited only with knee extension) is treated differently versus generalized Achilles contracture, both in therapy and surgery. Hindfoot alignment should also be documented, as a preexisting pes planovalgus deformity may increase after posterior tibial tendon transfer to the dorsal foot. Patients should be placed in a solid ankle foot orthosis and night splint to maintain passive dorsiflexion and to help facilitate walking.

Rehabilitation for the knee injury should also be considered; flexion contractures or limited knee range of motion may affect long-term walking potential, so these should also be addressed before consideration of posterior tibial tendon transfer. Weight loss

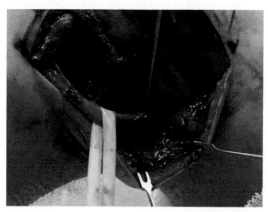

Fig. 2. Incomplete stretch injury to the CPN. (*Courtesy of* Mark Miller, MD, Charlottesville, VA.)

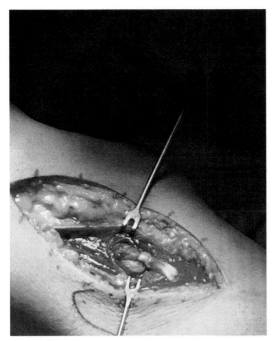

Fig. 3. Complete transection of the CPN. (*Courtesy of* Mark Miller, MD, Charlottesville, VA.)

in obese patients, as well as smoking cessation, may decrease the risk of possible surgical complications, including loss of tendon fixation/tension, wound complications, and infections.

Electromyography and nerve conduction studies are performed 6 weeks after the initial nerve injury. These results are then compared with a repeat study after an additional 6 weeks to document any changes that may occur. Specifically, motor nerve conduction studies of the common peroneal and tibial nerves are routinely performed, as well as sensory nerve conduction studies of the superficial peroneal, tibial and sural nerves.[13] Needle electromyography routinely tests 2 muscles innervated by the deep peroneal nerve, 1 muscle innervated by the superficial nerve, namely, the tibialis posterior (tibial nerve), an additional muscle innervated by the tibial nerve, and the short head of the biceps femoris. In the case of CPN injury owing to trauma, compound muscle action potentials will be decreased at all stimulation sites in the peroneal nerve distribution. If interval improvement is present, either clinically or on electromyography or nerve conduction studies, tendon transfer is typically delayed until 1 year after the injury.

SURGICAL CONSIDERATIONS

Once all nonoperative measures have been used, if a patient with persistent foot drop wishes to proceed with posterior tibial tendon transfer, the risks, benefits, and alternatives to surgery are discussed at length. The patient is informed that the surgery can eliminate or decrease dependence on an ankle-foot orthosis (AFO) brace for walking, and that it may improve hip and knee function owing to improved gait kinematics. A distal local anesthetic block for the surgical incision sites is preferred versus a sciatic or saphenous block given the known nerve injury pattern and potential for injury to the tibial branch of the sciatic nerve during popliteal block.

Preoperatively, if less than 10° of passive dorsiflexion is not obtainable, a Strayer procedure (for isolated gastrocnemius contracture) or tendo-Achilles lengthening is performed to achieve 10° of dorsiflexion. Given the inherent imbalance in plantarflexion strength and dorsiflexion strength, the posterior tibial tendon transfer cannot overcome an equinus contracture if it is not addressed surgically. Persistent equinus contracture will also make passage of the posterior tibial tendon into the lateral cuneiform bone tunnel exceedingly difficult. If a significant pes planovalgus deformity is present, a medial displacement calcaneal osteotomy and even flexor digitorum longus tendon transfer to the navicular tuberosity can be considered at the time of posterior tibial tendon transfer. However, functional loss of the posterior tibial tendon for inversion is less significant in CPN injuries, because it is balanced by the lack of dynamic eversion/peroneal tendon function (superficial peroneal nerve innervation).

SURGICAL TECHNIQUE

A medial midfoot incision is performed to expose the main posterior tibial tendon insertion onto the navciular tuberosity. The posterior tibial tendon is carefully elevated from the navicular tuberosity; including the periosteum and a portion of the accessory attachments of the posterior tibial tendon may provide additional length that can facilitate additional tendon to bone contact within the lateral cuneiform tunnel.

A more proximal medial incision is made along the posterior aspect of the medial malleolus and posterior tibia. The flexor retinaculum may need to be incised to allow for passage of the posterior tibial tendon into the proximal aspect of the medial ankle, and care should be taken to protect the neurovascular bundle inferiorly. The interosseus membrane is then bluntly opened using a curved clamp, hugging the posterior border of the tibia to avoid injury to the peroneal artery and vein, as well as the anterior tibial artery and deep peroneal nerve. A counter incision is then made at the distal one-third level of the tibia, over the lateral border of the tibia. The anterior compartment musculature should be bluntly elevated from the anterolateral tibia to visualize the clamp entering the tibia–fibula interval. Once this clamp can be clearly visualized, the clamp or periosteal elevator can be used to open an approximately 4-cm window in the interosseous membrane. If the intended passage is too distal, impingement with the syndesmotic ligaments and tibia–fibula overlap will prevent passage of the posterior tibial tendon.

After the tendon is recovered in the anterior aspect of the ankle, a running whip-stitch is placed into the posterior tibial tendon. The tendon is sized at this time, in preparation for passage and fixation of the tendon within the lateral cuneiform. The posterior tibial tendon is typically approximately 5 to 7 mm in diameter, after preparation and whip stitching.

After a fourth incision is made over the interval between the lateral cuneiform and cuboid, a guide wire is placed in a lateral to medial direction, centered in the lateral cuneiform and through the middle and medial cuneiforms. A dorsal to plantar tunnel can also be used, but requires a plantar incision in the foot, and less total cuneiform surface area when compared with the size of the bone tunnel. A smaller diameter hole (4.5 mm) is drilled across the 3 cuneiforms, followed by the appropriate tendon sized-hole (approximately 6.0 mm) drilled across the lateral cuneiform and a portion of the middle cuneiform. The ankle is then maximally dorsiflexed, and the tendon and sutures are passed through the bone tunnels in a lateral to medial direction. After direct visual confirmation that the tendon is well-situated within the lateral cuneiform, an interference screw is placed into the tunnel entrance. The whip stitch is then retrieved through the medial incision, and used to capture the tibialis anterior insertion and periosteum at the medial cuneiform. Appropriate tension and ankle position is confirmed, and the ankle is splinted in full dorsiflexion. Concomitant flexor digitorum longus transfer to the navicular can also be performed, which may help support the medial longitudinal arch and may improve balance and gait. **Fig. 4** demonstrates a schematic overview of the surgical procedure.

Postoperatively, the sutures are removed at 2 weeks, and the patient is placed into a short leg cast in maximal dorsiflexion for 4 weeks. The patient is permitted to begin ambulation in a boot at 6 weeks postoperatively, and begins active or active-assisted dorsiflexion with gradual progression of plantarflexion. The patient will begin formal physical therapy and is permitted to plantarflex to 10° below neutral and slowly progresses to 30° below neutral over the next 6 weeks. They are transitioned to a carbon fiber AFO at 3 months, and are asked to use a night splint to maintain dorsiflexion until 6 months postoperative. If preoperative therapy has been used to optimize the function of the posterior tibial tendon, recruitment and activation of the tendon transfer occurs early in the postoperative period.

At 6 months postoperative, all range of motion restrictions are lifted, and gradual progression to return-to-run protocols may be initiated. Cautious return to sports may occur at 9 months, although this is not the expectation or the goal of the surgery.

OUTCOMES

Although there are few studies examining the outcomes of the posterior tibial tendon transfer, most show good to excellent results. A 2016 study by Werner and colleagues[3] compared the functional outcomes of patients who underwent posterior tibial tendon transfer with patients who were treated with AFO only for CPN injury owing to a multiligament knee injury. They showed an increase in ankle dorsiflexion and eversion strength from 0 of 5 preoperatively to 4.75 of 5 and 4 of 5, respectively, in patients who underwent posterior tibial tendon transfer. Additionally, ankle motion improved from less than 0° of dorsiflexion preoperatively to 6.67° postoperatively. All 5 operative patients were able to ambulate without a brace at final follow-up. Gait analysis was also performed, which showed that patients treated nonoperatively required substantially more compensatory hip and knee flexion compared with the contralateral limb, which could result in long-term negative effects on adjacent joints, especially in patients recovering from an ipsilateral knee injury. Overall, patients who underwent posterior tibial tendon transfer showed gait patterns more similar to healthy controls but, as expected, did not correct all deficiencies. Balanced dynamic dorsiflexion resulting from posterior tibial tendon transfer is demonstrated in Video 1.

A similar study by Cho and colleagues[10] in 2017 corroborated these results. They showed a significant improvement in 3 distinct functional outcome measures (American Orthopaedic Foot and Ankle Society, Foot and Ankle Outcome Score, and Foot and Ankle Ability Measure) in patients who underwent posterior tibial tendon transfer compared with matched controls, despite dorsiflexion strength measuring 33% of normal. Additionally, there was a significant increase in dorsiflexion strength and range of motion, and only 1 in 17 required an AFO postoperatively for occupational activity. Molund and colleagues[14] also reported on a series of 12 patients who underwent posterior tibial tendon transfer; they showed a restoration of strength to 42% and of range of motion to 72% compared with the contralateral limb. Additionally, they report at least 4 patients who were able to maintain a high activity level, including a patient completing a marathon.

In 2014, Ho and colleagues[15] published their case series comparing delayed posterior tibial tendon transfer to the lateral cuneiform with early posterior tibial tendon

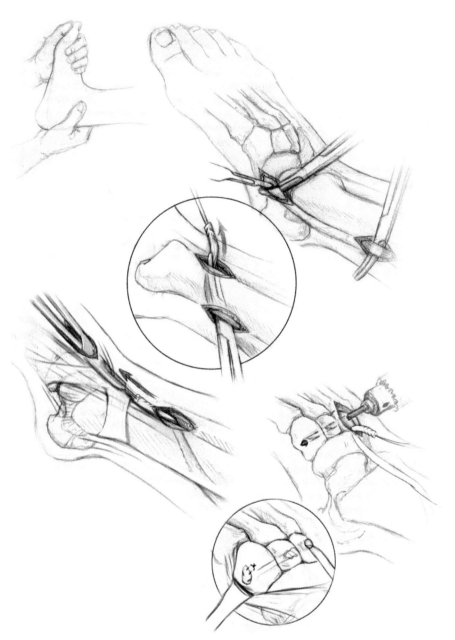

Fig. 4. Posterior tibial tendon transfer procedure. (*From* Werner BC, Norte GE, Hadeed MM, et al. Peroneal Nerve Dysfunction due to Multiligament Knee Injury: Patient Characteristics and Comparative Outcomes After Posterior Tibial Tendon Transfer. Clin J Sport Med. 2017 Jan;27(1):12; with permission.)

transfer in conjunction with CPN exploration/repair. For the early transfer/nerve repair group, 4 of 7 patients were able to return to running, with 2 returning to competitive sports. The authors proposed that earlier transfer may improve outcomes owing to avoidance of fixed equinus contracture and atrophy of the posterior tibial muscle/

tendon, and may have a beneficial effect on nerve regeneration after repair. They advocated for posterior tibial tendon transfer and CPN repair after 3 months in conjunction with flexor digitorum longus tendon transfer to the navicular, which could offset any possible return of function of the peroneal tendons.

The longest term follow-up (to the authors' knowledge) on outcomes after posterior tibial tendon transfer was reported by Yeap and colleagues[16] in 2001. They followed 12 patients who underwent posterior tibial tendon transfer for a mean of 90 months and found that 11 of the 12 patients were able to maintain 4 out of 5 or 5 out of 5 strength in ankle dorsiflexion despite only generating 30% of the torque (as measured on Cybex testing) of the uninjured limb. Additionally, 83% of patients rated their outcome as excellent or good, with the best outcomes in male patients under the age of 30%, and 83% of patient did not require an AFO postoperatively. Interestingly, although 4 of the 12 patients developed a flatter medial longitudinal arch after posterior tibial tendon transfer, none of these patients developed pain or symptoms consistent with an acquired flatfoot deformity. This finding is likely related to the absence of dynamic eversion owing to the functional loss of the peroneal tendons.

SUMMARY

Multiple studies show improved function in patients who underwent a posterior tibial tendon transfer compared with patients treated nonoperatively. For patients who develop a foot drop secondary to a CPN injury, posterior tibial tendon transfer should be considered when nonoperative measures fail and functional deficits persist. Early referral to a provider with experience in this procedure may improve patient satisfaction and patient reported outcomes after a knee dislocation or multiligament injury. In the future, additional large-scale or multicenter long-term outcomes studies are needed to confirm the promising results from the limited existing literature.

DISCLOSURE

The authors have no disclosures that are relevant to this article.

SUPPLEMENTARY DATA

Supplementary data related to this article can be found online at https://doi.org/10.1016/j.csm.2020.07.003.

REFERENCES

1. Rihn JA, Groff YJ, Harner CD, et al. The acutely dislocated knee: evaluation and management. J Am Acad Orthop Surg 2004;12:334–46.
2. Robertson A, Nutton RW, Keating JF. Dislocation of the knee. J Bone Joint Surg Br 2006;88:706–11.
3. Werner BC, Norte GE, Hadeed MM, et al. Peroneal nerve dysfunction due to multiligament knee injury: patient characteristics and comparative outcomes after posterior tibial tendon transfer. Clin J Sport Med 2017;27(1):10–9.
4. Arom GA, Yeranosian MG, Petrigliano FA, et al. The changing demographics of knee dislocation: a retrospective database review. Clin Orthop Relat Res 2014;472(9):2609–14.
5. Schenck RC Jr. The dislocated knee. Instr Course Lect 1994;43:127–36.
6. Moatshe G, Dornan GJ, Løken S, et al. Demographics and injuries associated with knee dislocation: a prospective review of 303 patients. Orthop J Sports Med 2017;5(5). 2325967117706521.

7. Keating JF. Acute knee ligament injuries and knee dislocation. In: Bentley G, editor. European surgical orthopaedics and traumatology. Berlin: Springer-Verlag GmbH; 2014. p. 2949–71.

8. Stewart RJ, Landy DC, Khazai RS, et al. Association of injury energy level and neurovascular injury following knee dislocation. J Orthop Trauma 2018;32(11): 579–84.

9. Krych AJ, Giuseffi SA, Kuzma SA, et al. Is peroneal nerve injury associated with worse function after knee dislocation? Clin Orthop Relat Res 2014;472(9):2630–6.

10. Cho BK, Park KJ, Choi SM, et al. Functional outcomes following anterior transfer of the tibialis posterior tendon for foot drop secondary to peroneal nerve palsy. Foot Ankle Int 2017;38(6):627–33.

11. Wagner E, Wagner P, Zanolli D, et al. Biomechanical evaluation of circumtibial and transmembranous routes for posterior tibial tendon transfer for dropfoot. Foot Ankle Int 2018;39(7):843–9.

12. Coughlin MJ, Mann RA, Saltzman CL. Surgery of the foot and ankle. 8th edition. Philadelphia: Mosby-Elsevier; 2007.

13. Baima J, Krivickas L. Evaluation and treatment of peroneal neuropathy. Curr Rev Musculoskelet Med 2008;1(2):147–53.

14. Molund M, Engebretsen L, Hvaal K, et al. Posterior tibial tendon transfer improves function for foot drop after knee dislocation. Clin Orthop Relat Res 2014. https://doi.org/10.1007/s11999-014-3533-x.

15. Ho B, Khan Z, Switaj PJ, et al. Treatment of peroneal nerve injuries with simultaneous tendon transfer and nerve exploration. J Orthop Surg Res 2014;9:67.

16. Yeap JS, Birch R, Singh D. Long-term results of tibialis posterior tendon transfer for drop-foot. Int Orthop 2001;25(2):114–8.

Chronic Lateral Ankle Instability: Surgical Management

Eric Ferkel, MD*, Shawn Nguyen, DO, Cory Kwong, MD

KEYWORDS

- Chronic lateral ankle instability • Modified Broström procedure
- Arthroscopic treatment of lateral ankle ligament instability
- Suture tape augmentation for lateral ankle ligament instability

KEY POINTS

- Chronic ankle sprains with failure of nonoperative treatment lead to chronic lateral ankle instability (CLAI).
- Multiple surgical reconstruction techniques have been described for CLAI.
- The current recommendation is for open anatomic repair/reconstructions.
- Suture tape augmentation and arthroscopic Broström technique show a great deal of promise, with more research needed.

INTRODUCTION

Ankle sprains are one of the most common presenting complaints to musculoskeletal practitioners. There are more than 300,000 new cases of ankle sprains every year, with approximately 15% of them being classified as severe.[1] These injuries most commonly affect the lateral soft tissue structures of the ankle.

Most acute ankle sprains can be treated successfully with conservative measures, including rest, icing, antiinflammatory use, bracing, and progressive weight bearing in addition to physical therapy. However, recurrent ankle sprains can lead to chronic lateral ankle instability (CLAI) and significant functional impairment, especially in the athletic population; this can result in chronic pain, peroneal tendon injury, and risk of osteochondral injury to the talus.[2] It is also important to note that chronic ankle instability may develop in 20% to 30% of individuals despite adequate nonoperative management.[3]

The initial treatment of chronic ankle instability is a structured program of functional and prophylactic rehabilitation. Surgical intervention is indicated if rehabilitation fails to restore structural and functional ankle stability. This article focuses on surgical options

Southern California Orthopedic Institute, 6815 Noble Avenue, Suite 200, Van Nuys, CA 91405, USA
* Corresponding author.
E-mail address: eferkel@scoi.com

Clin Sports Med 39 (2020) 829–843
https://doi.org/10.1016/j.csm.2020.07.004
0278-5919/20/© 2020 Elsevier Inc. All rights reserved.

for the treatment of CLAI and includes a review of arthroscopic and open procedures as well as both anatomic and nonanatomic reconstructions to address CLAI.

NONANATOMIC RECONSTRUCTION

Initial attempts at restoring lateral ankle stability used the adjacent anatomy to substitute for a torn or attenuated anterior talofibular ligament (ATFL) and calcaneofibular ligament (CFL). In general, these procedures took the form of local tendon transfers of the peronei to constrain the lateral ankle. Because of inferior outcomes and higher complication rates associated with these techniques, they have largely been replaced by anatomic repair and reconstructive techniques.[4–6]

The Watson-Jones procedure was one of the first described reconstructive technique of the lateral ligamentous complex. In the original description, the peroneus brevis tendon was released proximally, then rerouted through the distal fibula and secured to the anterolateral talus and calcaneus.[1] Subsequent modifications of the procedure included harvesting part or the entirety of the peroneus longus tendon.[7] Initial outcomes were promising, with high rates of good and excellent results in several cohorts.[7,8] However, drawbacks of the procedure, including sural nerve injury, persistent calf asymmetry, loss of dynamic eversion strength, and incomplete restoration of ankle biomechanics, became more apparent comparing with the anatomic Broström.[9,10]

Other variations of peroneal tenodesis included the Evans and Chrisman-Snook. Evans abbreviated the Watson-Jones by simply passing the proximal aspect of the peroneus brevis tendon through the distal fibula. However, long-term outcomes were poor, with only 50% of patients reporting satisfactory results at an average of 14 years.[11]

The Chrisman-Snook procedure was a more elaborate tenodesis that used a split peroneus brevis graft passed anterior to posterior through the distal fibula and then proximal to distal through the lateral calcaneus and back onto itself to reconstruct both the ATFL and CFL.[12] Based on their long-term outcomes, Snook and colleagues[5] touted the procedure to be effective in a high percentage of patients. However, there was a high rate of lateral-sided numbness in the cohort, with 4 of 14 sural nerve injuries resulting in permanent deficits. In 1996, Hennrikus and colleagues[13] compared the Chrisman-Snook with the modified Broström in a randomized trial. They affirmed that the Chrisman-Snook could be effective at restoring lateral ankle stability but was inferior to the modified Broström in Sefton scores and complication rates.

Despite nonanatomic procedures being supplanted by anatomic approaches, their use may still be considered in the setting of complex hindfoot reconstruction or arthroplasty with concomitant instability.[14] Thus, an understanding of these procedures and their respective limitations remains important to a comprehensive understanding of the available surgical options.

OPEN ANATOMIC REPAIR

The shortcomings of nonanatomic repairs led to increasing interest in more anatomic procedures. The aim of these anatomic approaches was to restore the natural anatomy and biomechanics of the lateral ankle without compromising the adjacent structures and function of the ankle and subtalar joint.[15] The first anatomic approach to repair of the lateral ligaments was reported by Broström[16] in 1966. In this true anatomic method, the native lateral ligaments are isolated and repaired with a suture construct.[16] In many cases, the procedure proved more challenging to perform than initially described because the ligaments were often difficult to locate and of poor tissue quality.[13] In order to address the technical challenges of the original procedure, 2 main modifications were described by Karlsson and colleagues[11] and Gould.[17]

Karlsson and colleagues[11] described shortening the attenuated ATFL and CFL by repairing the distal portion of the ligaments directly to bone via drill holes in their anatomic positions on the distal fibula. The proximal ligament remnant and capsule was then imbricated over the repair. This approach avoided direct end-to-end suture repair while correcting for chronically elongated lateral tissues. In their original series of 92 ankles, 60% and 27% of patients had excellent and good outcomes, respectively. Of 20 patients with an unsatisfactory result, 16 were in patients with generalized hypermobility, long-standing ligamentous insufficiency, or previous tenodesis surgery. The investigators concluded that their anatomic repair produced good functional and mechanical results but was contraindicated in patients with the aforementioned risk factors.[11]

The Gould modification augmented the Broström repair with inclusion of the inferior extensor retinaculum, a technique that was coined the modified Broström procedure. Like other anatomic repairs, the ability to achieve a robust repair relies on the existing tissue quality.[15] In a cadaveric study, Aydogan and colleagues[18] found that the Gould modification took significantly more inversion force before failure than cadaveric specimens with a Broström-only repair. Subsequent cadaveric studies concluded that the additional stability provided by the modification is marginal.[19] Despite a lack of comparative clinical trials of the Broström to modified Broström, the modified Broström has largely become regarded as the initial treatment of choice for CLAI.[19,20]

Authors' Preferred Technique

The authors' preferred technique for anatomic repair is an anchorless Broström-Gould, which has been previously described.[15] In summary, an ankle arthroscopy is performed and all intra-articular disorder is addressed. Attention is then turned to the lateral ligaments. A curvilinear incision is used extending from the center of the distal fibula toward the sinus tarsi. This incision allows for anterior and posterior exposure and possible extension to evaluate and treat peroneal tendon disorder. Full-thickness flaps are developed to expose the ligaments, extensor retinaculum, and peroneal tendon sheath. It is imperative to stay superficial to the level of the extensor retinaculum to ensure that enough tissue is preserved to perform the Gould modification, which can be ensured by bluntly dissection anteriorly over the retinaculum with a small key elevator. The peroneal tendons are then exposed and inspected through a small oblique incision in the inferior peroneal sheath just posterior to the peroneal tendons. Any tenosynovitis or other disorder can be addressed at this time by extending the incision proximally or distally. The inferior extensor retinaculum is then mobilized and retracted. It is critical to identify the so-called soft-spot triangle between the ATFL and syndesmosis as the most proximal aspect of the arthrotomy. This triangle is appreciated as the soft spot between the origins of both ligaments on the fibula and can be easily penetrated with a small clamp (**Fig. 1**). With the inferior retinaculum retracted distally and the peroneal tendons protected with a Ragnell retractor, the ligaments are transected in an oblique fashion leaving a 2-mm to 3-mm cuff of tissue at the distal fibula for later repair. The capsuloligamentous tissue is then released distally and posteriorly to the level of the peroneal tendon sheath. The lateral talar dome and lateral gutter are inspected and the joint irrigated (**Fig. 2**).

The ATFL and CFL are then repaired at this time with the ankle maintained in a reduced position in slight eversion and neutral dorsiflexion with a bump behind the calf producing a posterior drawer; the sutures are then tied in a so-called pants-over-vest fashion from posterior to anterior (**Fig. 3**). If there is a concern for inadequate

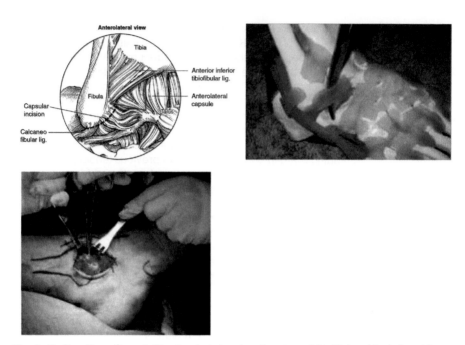

Fig. 1. Finding the soft spot. (Anatomical drawing Courtesy of Dr. Richard Ferkel and Susan Brust.)

soft tissue quality, suture anchors placed into the anatomic origins of the ATFL and CFL can be used to augment the reconstruction and allow for direct ligament to bone healing. If planning on using suture anchors with drill holes, it is preferred to perform ligament transection typically more proximal (directly off the tip of the fibula), in order to allow for tissue-to-bone healing. In cases of a distal fibular exostosis or

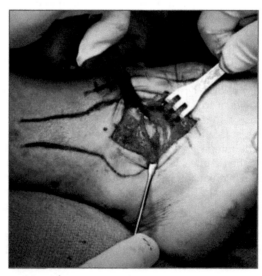

Fig. 2. Capsuloligamentous release.

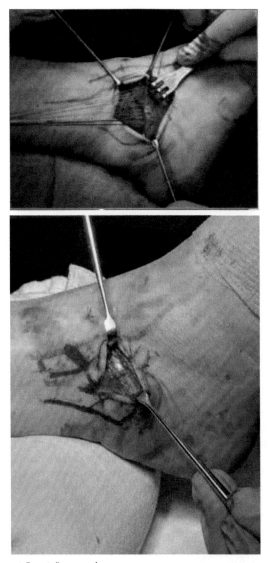

Fig. 3. Pants-over-vest Broström repair.

loose body from a prior avulsion, the use of suture anchors may allow a more reproducible method of fixation.

The peroneal sheath is repaired, and the inferior retinaculum is then imbricated to the periosteum of the distal fibula in a similar pants-over-vest technique to complete the Gould modification (**Fig. 4**). The wound is irrigated and closed, and a plaster splint is applied.[15,21]

In 2007, Ferkel and Chams[21] reported on their findings and long-term results after the aforementioned technique for CLAI combined with arthroscopic evaluation. Ninety-five percent of patients had associated intra-articular disorder, of which only 20% were apparent on open inspection via lateral arthrotomy. The most common

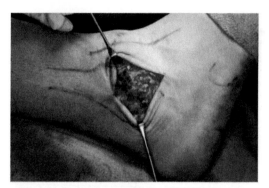

Fig. 4. Retinacular closure advancement, Gould modification.

disorder consisted of synovitis, adhesions, and chondromalacia. In this small retrospective series, all patients had excellent or good outcomes, 57% and 43%, respectively. The mean American Orthopaedic Foot and Ankle Society (AOFAS) ankle/hindfoot score was 97.1 at an average 60-month follow-up.[21]

Several other investigators have reported excellent long-term outcomes following the Broström and Broström-Gould procedures. In 2006, Bell and colleagues[22] reported their 26-year Broström outcomes in a Naval Academy cohort. Twenty-two patients had complete follow-up, of which 91% reported good or excellent ankle function with a mean Foot and Ankle Outcome Score (FAOS), as described by Roos1, of 92.[23] No radiographic or clinical outcomes were reported. Tourné and colleagues[24] reported long-term outcomes of the modified Broström-Gould, with 11 years of clinical follow-up. Their large multicenter retrospective study included 150 cases of lateral ankle instability and yielded 93% satisfactory results with no significant development of tibiotalar arthrosis.[24]

Return to play after lateral ligament reconstruction is of particular importance in the athletic population. The modified Broström has shown excellent results in elite and professional athletes. White and colleagues[25] performed the procedure on 42 professional athletes, all of whom returned to preinjury level and showed a mean return to sport of only 77 days. Lee and colleagues[26] also recently reported a 100% return to play in elite athletes, albeit with a more conservative timeline mean for return to competitive play of 3.9 months. Despite expedient return to play in the athletic population, further efforts have been dedicated to accelerating rehabilitation in the form of additional repair augmentation.

ALLOGRAFT RECONSTRUCTION

In patients with severe chronic ankle instability, failed primary repair, poor-quality remnant lateral ligaments, or high body mass index (BMI), reconstruction augmentation with autograft or allograft tissue is a suitable option for stabilization. Although autograft carries the advantage of decreased cost and eliminates the risk of disease transmission, allograft eliminates donor-site morbidity and may decrease surgical time, postoperative pain, and long-term mobility, especially in athletes. Numerous studies have been performed comparing the outcomes of allograft versus autograft reconstruction for CLAI and they have shown no difference in outcomes and complications.[27–30] Because of these findings, allograft augmentation has become increasingly popular for treating patients with CLAI, which may be especially relevant in patients with generalized ligamentous laxity or known connective tissue disorders where autograft tissue may be inadequate for reconstructive procedures.

In 2014, Jung and colleagues[28] reported on a large cohort of 70 patients treated with allograft reconstruction. Allograft reconstruction resulted in significant improvements in visual analog scale (VAS) pain scores (decreased from 5.5 to 1.3) and AOFAS scores (improved from 71 to 90.9). Their mean Karlsson-Peterson score also improved from 55.1 to 90.3 and the talar tilt decreased from 14.8° to 3.9°. Note that their technique did not include a repair of the native ligaments, unlike the technique later described by Dierckman and Ferkel.[31]

Li and colleagues[32] recently performed a systematic review and meta-analysis of outcomes after allograft reconstruction in patients with CLAI. They included 153 patients from 6 studies with an average follow-up duration of 34 months. The average AOFAS scores improved from 55.4 to 91.9, which was a 40% improvement. The pooled proportion of patients who returned to sports after surgery was 80%. The pooled total risk of recurrent instability after surgery was only 6%. In addition, no graft rejection was reported in any of the studies.

Dierckman and Ferkel[31] reported the results of this technique on 31 patients. They found that 20% of patients with CLAI required allograft augmentation in addition to a direct primary repair.

In their retrospective review, 100% of patients were completely satisfied at an average follow-up of 38 months. Their AOFAS ankle-hindfoot scores significantly improved from an average of 60.3 to 87.5. VAS pain scores significantly decreased from 7.3 to 1.9. On follow-up stress radiographs, the mean talar tilt decreased from 14.3° to 3.1°. Note that no patients developed arthritic changes beyond grade 1 on plain radiographs.

Authors' Preferred Technique

The indications listed in **Box 1** describe when the authors decide to use the allograft anatomic reconstruction technique to address chronic lateral ankle ligament instability.

Briefly, a fresh-frozen, nonirradiated semitendinosus allograft is used to anatomically recreate both the ATFL and CFL. In the absence of generalized ligamentous laxity or connective tissue disorder, autograft hamstring can also be used. Before the open procedure, a standard ankle arthroscopy is performed and all concomitant intra-articular disorder is addressed. The reconstruction uses a similar approach to the anatomic Broström procedure described earlier. The anatomic

---

Box 1
Indications for using a semitendinosus allograft to correct lateral ankle instability

Indications
- Significant ankle laxity with greater than 10° difference in talar tilt angle compared with the opposite side or an absolute talar tilt angle greater than 15°
- Previously failed reconstruction of the lateral ligaments
- Generalized ligamentous laxity
- Obesity (BMI>30 kg/m^2)
- High-demand heavy athletes or laborers
- Poor-quality tissue during the intraoperative evaluation

Reconstruction with a semitendinosus allograft was performed on any patient having more than 2 of the criteria listed.

From Dierckman BD, Ferkel RD. Anatomic Reconstruction with a Semitendinosus Allograft for Chronic Lateral Ankle Instability. *Am J Sports Med.* 2015;43(8):1941-1950.; with permission.

insertion of the ATFL on the lateral talar neck is exposed. A guidewire is inserted at the insertion approximately 18 mm proximal to the subtalar joint. The guidewire is then overdrilled to a depth of 20 mm, usually with a 5.5-mm diameter drill. Next, the distal fibula is exposed and a guide pin is inserted in an anterior-to-posterior direction beginning at the ATFL origin. A tunnel is then created by drilling over the guide pin to the posterior aspect of the fibula. A second guidewire is then inserted at the distal tip of the fibula to converge near the exit of the previously drilled tunnel, taking care to maintain a posterior bone bridge between the ATFL and CFL tunnels. Intersection of the tunnels within the fibula may increase the risk of gradual loosening of the respective limbs because of displacement of cancellous bone. Alternatively, the ATFL limb may be angled more proximal posterior to allow for a larger bony bridge between the 2 tunnels if there is concern of tunnel enlargement in poor-quality bone.

The 2 tunnels are overdrilled, usually up to 5 mm, to create 2 tunnels from the ATFL origin to the posterior fibula, and from the posterior fibula to the CFL origin. Care is taken to ensure the sockets are drilled in the center of the fibula to avoid tunnel blowout. The tendon graft is first secured into the talar neck tunnel with a biotenodesis-type screw, then passed through the ATFL and CFL tunnels respectively.

To secure the CFL limb into the calcaneus, a point is marked on the skin approximately 13 mm inferior to the subtalar joint at an angle of 130° from the fibular shaft. A stab incision is made and blunt dissection performed to the calcaneus, and a guide pin is inserted at this level from lateral to medial with care taken to avoid the neurovascular bundle at the medial exit point. The appropriately sized cannulated drill is advanced over the guide pin in a lateral-to-medial direction. The graft is tunneled from the fibula, under the peroneal tendons, and delivered out the calcaneal incision. Subsequently, the suture tails and any remaining graft are delivered out the medial heel using the eyelet on the guide pin (**Fig. 5**).

The ankle is placed in 0° of dorsiflexion and slight eversion, and a posterior drawer is applied to the ankle while the graft is secured with interference screw fixation into the tunnel. Care must be taken to apply appropriate tension to the graft, ensuring adequate tension of both ATFL and CFL limbs (**Fig. 6**). A modified Broström is then performed over the top with the remnant tissue.

Based on the amount of literature published on allograft reconstruction in patients with CLAI, this procedure has resulted in significant improvements in patient function and outcome scores, with low rates of recurrent instability. Moreover, allograft usage avoids the risk of donor-site morbidity and with faster surgical times and a low complication rate.

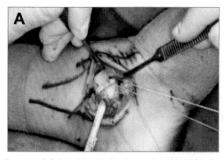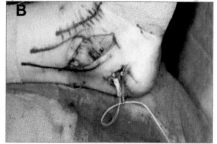

Figs. 5. (*A*) Passing the allograft through the fibula. (*B*) Passing the allograft through the calcaneus to secure the CFL limb.

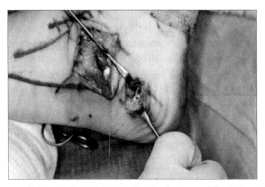

Fig. 6. Final construct of allograft augmentation before modified Broström closure.

LATERAL ANKLE LIGAMENT REPAIR WITH SUTURE TAPE AUGMENTATION

A newly evolving technique in the treatment of CLAI is ligament tape augmentation. The nonabsorbable suture tape is typically made with a combination of high-molecular-weight polyethylene and polyester and is produced by various manufacturers. There are several suture tape augmentation techniques, which consist of performing a modified Broström procedure followed by knotless anchor insertion of a suture tape construct[33–36] (**Fig. 7**).

The possible advantages of this augmentation are to provide a strong checkrein of the native ligament repair, and also to allow for early mobilization and maybe allow for rehabilitation before the biological healing of the native repair is completed. In addition, there are early data to show it may provide greater strength when there is poor ligamentous tissue quality and in cases of generalized ligamentous laxity, patients with high BMI, and elite athletes.

There have been biomechanical studies that show the strength of suture tape. In a recent study, Viens and colleagues[35] compared suture tape augmentation to Broström repair with suture tape augmentation to an intact ATFL. Based on their results

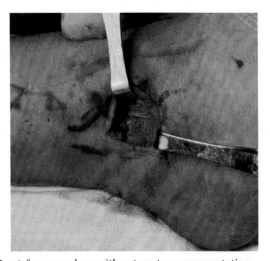

Fig. 7. Modified Broström procedure with suture tape augmentation.

from fresh-frozen cadavers, the mean ultimate load to failure of suture tape augmentation was significantly higher than that of the intact ATFL (315 vs 154 N) and there was no difference between the Broström repair with suture tape augmentation and intact ATFL. The mean stiffness of the Broström repair with augmentation was similar to the native ATFL. However, this study could not account for ultimate biological healing, only initial biomechanical stability. In a second biomechanical study, Schuh and colleagues[34] compared the torsional stability of the traditional Broström repair, Broström repair with suture anchors, and Broström repair with tape augmentation. They evaluated the angle at which the ankle failed, and the ATFL reconstruction failed at 24.1°, the suture anchor group failed at 35.5°, and the internal brace group failed at 46.9° ($P = .02$). In addition, torque at failure reached 5.7 Nm for the Broström group, 8.0 Nm for the suture anchor repair, and 11.2 Nm for the tape augmentation group ($P = .04$), showing statistically significant additive biomechanical advantage supporting the use of suture anchors as well as tape augmentation.

Cho and colleagues[33] were among the first to describe the clinical results of suture tape augmentation for CLAI. They reviewed a case series of 34 young female patients with less than 70 kg body weight with 2-year follow-up. The average subjective satisfaction score was 93.8. Talar tilt and anterior talar translation significantly improved an average of 4.5° and 4.1 mm, respectively. According to the Sefton grading, 91% of the patients achieved satisfactory functional results. At final follow-up, the mean foot and ankle outcome scores improved from an average of 63.1 preoperatively to 93.2 ($P = .001$).

A recent study on this technique published by Xu and colleagues[36] compared modified Broström repairs with and without suture tape augmentation, with at least 2-year follow-up. This study included 25 patients undergoing modified Broström repair with suture tape augmentation and 28 patients with isolated modified Broström repair. Both groups achieved satisfactory outcomes and significant improvements in terms of pain and functional outcome scores. There were no statistical differences between the 2 groups when comparing range of motion, VAS, AOFAS scores, and radiologic outcomes. However, when comparing the Foot and Ankle Ability Measure surveys, the suture tape augmentation group had significantly better scores than the isolated Broström repair for the sport (87.1 vs 78.2) and total (93.1 vs 90.5) outcome surveys.

Suture tape augmentation of the ATFL repair has the potential to allow early weight bearing and ankle motion, limit immobilization time, and allow a quicker return to function. However, it must be performed as an augmentation to modified Broström repair, to ensure biological ligamentous healing, and it is imperative to not overtension the suture tape during its placement The suture tape is not a replacement for the Broström procedure but an augmentation that, although a promising technique, requires further research to be performed in order to prove its full utility and effectiveness.

ROLE OF ARTHROSCOPY

As ankle arthroscopy has evolved, its main indication for use in treating the unstable ankle was to aid in diagnosing concomitant ankle disorders that could potentially be overlooked preoperatively. These intra-articular conditions associated with CLAI include impingement, loose bodies, osteochondral lesions, chondromalacia, and bone spurs.[15,21,37] These injuries can lead to devastating long-term effects if left untreated despite surgical stabilization of the lateral ankle ligaments. Komenda and Ferkel's[38] study involved performing diagnostic ankle arthroscopy on 55 ankles with chronic instability. The investigators found that 93% of their patients had associated lesions requiring intervention that were only diagnosed through arthroscopy and not seen on preoperative imaging. Disorders included osteochondral lesions of the talus, synovitis, ossicles, and osteophytes. With treatment of these injuries in addition to the chronic ankle instability, 96% of the patients experienced good to excellent results.

A more recent study by Staats and colleagues[39] was designed to determine the reliability and validity of preoperative MRI and the detection of additional disorders in patients with CLAI. A group of 30 patients was studied, and, through the routine use of arthroscopy, the investigators were able to find 72 disorders in addition to the 73 that were appreciated on preoperative MRI.

As techniques of ankle arthroscopy have advanced, so has its usefulness to address various ankle disorders, including ligament instability. In addition to its diagnostic purposes, definitive therapeutic procedures have been undertaken. Arthroscopic thermal stabilization has been described in the treatment CLAI.[40–42] Similar to the treatment of shoulder laxity, thermal capsular shrinkage works by denaturing the collagen molecules within the capsule using electrocautery, resulting in tightening of the capsule through the reparative process. The original notion was that thermal capsular shrinkage in the ankle would have better results than in the shoulder because of the inherent stability of the ankle mortise. Maiotti and colleagues[42] retrospectively reviewed 22 soccer players with CLAI and treated them with arthroscopic thermal capsular shrinkage. At an average follow-up of 42 months, the investigators reported good or excellent functional outcomes with no evidence of ankle instability in 86% of their cohort.

Even with the popularity and success of open ATFL repair, interest has increased in the use of an arthroscopic Broström repair technique. The first surgeons to describe the arthroscopic ATFL repair were Hawkins[43] and Ferkel and Scranton[44] in the 1990s. Similar to many novel procedures, the initial learning period was associated with too many complications and longer surgical times compared with the open procedures. However, with the advancements and development of arthroscopic instruments and techniques related to ankle surgery, arthroscopic ATFL repair has become more popular. Acevedo and Mangone[45] have led the modern development of arthroscopic lateral ankle ligament reconstructions and recently defined a safe zone at 1.5 cm from the fibular tip to avoid the intermediate branch of the superficial peroneal nerve. The publication of this arthroscopic safe zone can assist surgeons in avoiding a nerve injury (**Fig. 8**).

Brown and colleagues[46] performed a systematic review in 2018 on arthroscopic repair of the lateral ankle ligaments, which included 8 studies for a total of 269 ankles. They concluded that arthroscopic repair was effective in improving AOFAS scores on an average of 22.8 to 54.2 points with an average follow-up of 17 months. In addition, the complication rate was 11.6% and the overall rate of return to sport was 100%. However, Matsui and colleagues[47] performed a recent systematic review comparing open and arthroscopic repairs and found that, based on the lack of quality evidence, they did not recommend the use of arthroscopic repair. Yeo and colleagues[48] performed a randomized trial comparing open versus arthroscopic repair on 48 patients and concluded that there was no difference in clinical or radiographic outcomes at 1 year after surgery.

The most recent advancement of arthroscopic lateral ankle stabilization was the use of allograft reconstruction. In 2018, Lopes and colleagues[49] published a prospective study comparing arthroscopic ATFL repair and gracilis allograft reconstruction. They included a total of 286 patients, with 115 undergoing repair and 171 with reconstruction. Both procedures resulted in significant improvement in AOFAS (62.1 preoperatively to 89.2 postoperatively) and Karlsson scores (55 to 87.1). These scores were not significantly different between the groups treated by repair and by reconstruction.

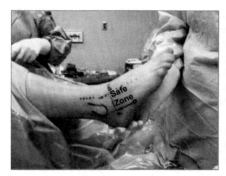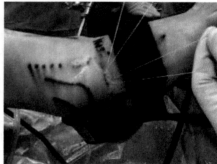

Fig. 8. Arthroscopic lateral ankle ligament reconstruction. (*Courtesy of* Jorge Acevedo, MD and Pete Mangone, MD.)

The role of arthroscopy in chronic lateral instability has grown since its first use nearly 3 decades ago. From thermal capsular shrinkage to anatomic arthroscopic repair and reconstruction, the leaders of ankle arthroscopy are pushing the envelope on the capabilities of minimally invasive surgery. The benefits of minimal incisions and quicker rehabilitation may outweigh any longer surgical time, steeper learning curve, and higher neurologic complication rate. Although arthroscopic Broström repair procedures are increasing in popularity, further studies need to be performed to show its true effectiveness and advantages compared with similar open procedures.

SUMMARY

Through decades of advancement in the treatment of chronic lateral ankle ligament instability, many techniques have been described and advocated. Anatomic, nonanatomic, allograft, suture tape augmentation, and arthroscopic techniques are all discussed in this article. However, the gold standard at this time remains the open anatomic Broström repair with the Gould augmentation with early range of motion and limited immobilization. The addition of strength with suture tape augmentation, and the minimal invasive approach of the all-arthroscopic and the allograft techniques, all have advantages and disadvantages and, when appropriately indicated, can safely lead to a successful outcome. However, greater research still must be done to provide the safest and most efficacious combination of procedures to provide patients with the best outcomes.

DISCLOSURE

Dr E. Ferkel discloses that he is a consultant and instructor for Arthrex and Ferring Pharmaceuticals. Dr S. Nguyen and C. Kwong have nothing to disclose. Southern California Orthopedic Institute Sports Medicine and Arthroscopy Fellowship receives institutional support from Depuy Mitek and Smith & Nephew.

REFERENCES

1. Ferran NA, Oliva F, Maffulli N. Ankle instability. Sports Med Arthrosc Rev 2009; 17(2):139–45.
2. Maffulli N, Ferran NA. Management of acute and chronic ankle instability. J Am Acad Orthop Surg 2008;16(10):608–15.

3. Hertel J. Functional anatomy, pathomechanics, and pathophysiology of lateral ankle instability. J Athl Train 2002;37(4):364–75.
4. Krips R, van Dijk CN, Lehtonen H, et al. Sports activity level after surgical treatment for chronic anterolateral ankle instability: a multicenter study. Am J Sports Med 2002;30(1):13–9.
5. Snook GA, Chrisman OD, Wilson TC. Long-term results of the Chrisman-Snook operation for reconstruction of the lateral ligaments of the ankle. J Bone Joint Surg Am 1985;67(1):1–7.
6. Krips R, van Dijk CN, Halasi T, et al. Anatomical reconstruction versus tenodesis for the treatment of chronic anterolateral instability of the ankle joint: a 2- to 10-year follow-up, multicenter study. Knee Surg Sports Traumatol Arthrosc 2000; 8(3):173–9.
7. Barbari SG, Brevig K, Egge T. Reconstruction of the lateral ligamentous structures of the ankle with a modified watson-jones procedure. Foot Ankle 1987; 7(6):362–8.
8. Younes C, Fowles JV, Fallaha M, et al. Long-term results of surgical reconstruction for chronic lateral instability of the ankle: comparison of Watson-Jones and Evans techniques. J Trauma 1988;28(9):1330–4.
9. Sugimoto K, Takakura Y, Akiyama K, et al. Long-term results of watson-jones tenodesis of the ankle. clinical and radiographic findings after ten to eighteen years of follow-up. J Bone Joint Surg Am 1998;80(11):1587–96.
10. Bahr R, Pena F, Shine J, et al. Biomechanics of ankle ligament reconstruction: an in vitro comparison of the broström repair, watson-jones reconstruction, and a new anatomic reconstruction technique. Am J Sports Med 1997;25(4):424–32.
11. Karlsson J, Bergsten T, Lansinger O, et al. Lateral instability of the ankle treated by the Evans procedure. A long-term clinical and radiological follow-up. J Bone Joint Surg Br 1988;70-B(3):476–80.
12. Chrisman O, Snook G. Reconstruction of lateral ligament tears of the ankle: an experimental study and clinical evaluation of seven patients treated by a new modification of the elmslie procedure. J Bone Joint Surg Am 1969;51(5):904–12.
13. Hennrikus WL, Mapes RC, Lyons PM, et al. Outcomes of the chrisman-snook and modified-broström procedures for chronic lateral ankle instability: a prospective, randomized comparison. Am J Sports Med 1996;24(4):400–4.
14. Yasui Y, Shimozono Y, Kennedy JG. Surgical procedures for chronic lateral ankle instability. J Am Acad Orthop Surg 2018;26(7):223–30.
15. Ferkel RD. Foot & ankle arthroscopy. 2nd edition. Philadelphia: Wolters Kluwer; 2017.
16. Broström L. Sprained ankles. VI. Surgical treatment of "chronic" ligament ruptures. Acta Chir Scand 1966;132(5):551–65.
17. Gould N, Seligson D, Gassman J. Early and late repair of lateral ligament of the ankle. Foot & ankle 1980;1(2):84–9.
18. Aydogan U, Glisson R, Nunley J. Extensor retinaculum augmentation reinforces anterior talofibular ligament repair. Clin Orthop 2006;442:210–5.
19. Behrens SB, Drakos M, Lee BJ, et al. Biomechanical analysis of broström versus broström-gould lateral ankle instability repairs. Foot Ankle Int 2013;34(4):587–92.
20. Porter M, Shadbolt B, Ye X, et al. Ankle lateral ligament augmentation versus the modified broström-gould procedure: a 5-year randomized controlled trial. Am J Sports Med 2019;47(3):659–66.
21. Ferkel RD, Chams RN. Chronic lateral instability: arthroscopic findings and long-term results. Foot Ankle Int 2007;28(1):24–31.

22. Bell SJ, Mologne TS, Sitler DF, et al. Twenty-six-year results after Broström procedure for chronic lateral ankle instability. The American journal of sports medicine 2006;34(6):975–8.

23. Roos EM, Brandsson S, Karlsson J. Validation of the foot and ankle outcome score for ankle ligament reconstruction. Foot Ankle Int 2001;22:788–94.

24. Tourné Y, Mabit C, Moroney PJ, et al. Long-term follow-up of lateral reconstruction with extensor retinaculum flap for chronic ankle instability. Foot Ankle Int 2012; 33(12):1079–86.

25. White WJ, McCollum GA, Calder JDF. Return to sport following acute lateral ligament repair of the ankle in professional athletes. Knee Surg Sports Traumatol Arthrosc 2016;24(4):1124–9.

26. Lee K, Jegal H, Chung H, et al. Return to play after modified Broström operation for chronic ankle instability in elite athletes. Clinics in Orthopedic Surgery 2019; 11(1):126–30.

27. Yasui Y, Murawski CD, Wollstein A, et al. Operative Treatment of Lateral Ankle Instability. JBJS Rev 2016;4(5). https://doi.org/10.2106/JBJS.RVW.15.00074.

28. Jung H-G, Shin M-H, Park J-T, et al. Anatomical reconstruction of lateral ankle ligaments using free tendon allografts and biotenodesis screws. Foot Ankle Int 2015;36(9):1064–71.

29. Xu X, Hu M, Liu J, et al. Minimally invasive reconstruction of the lateral ankle ligaments using semitendinosus autograft or tendon allograft. Foot Ankle Int 2014; 35(10):1015–21.

30. Matheny LM, Johnson NS, Liechti DJ, et al. Activity level and function after lateral ankle ligament repair versus reconstruction. Am J Sports Med 2016;44(5): 1301–8.

31. Dierckman BD, Ferkel RD. Anatomic Reconstruction with a Semitendinosus Allograft for Chronic Lateral Ankle Instability. Am J Sports Med 2015;43(8):1941–50.

32. Li H, Song Y, Li H, et al. Outcomes after anatomic lateral ankle ligament reconstruction using allograft tendon for chronic ankle instability: a systematic review and meta-analysis. J Foot Ankle Surg 2020;59(1):117–24.

33. Cho B-K, Park K-J, Kim S-W, et al. Minimal invasive suture-tape augmentation for chronic ankle instability. Foot Ankle Int 2015;36(11):1330–8.

34. Schuh R, Benca E, Willegger M, et al. Comparison of Broström technique, suture anchor repair, and tape augmentation for reconstruction of the anterior talofibular ligament. Knee Surg Sports Traumatol Arthrosc 2016;24(4):1101–7.

35. Viens NA, Wijdicks CA, Campbell KJ, et al. Anterior talofibular ligament ruptures, part 1: biomechanical comparison of augmented Broström repair techniques with the intact anterior talofibular ligament. Am J Sports Med 2014;42(2):405–11.

36. Xu D-L, Gan K-F, Li H-J, et al. Modified Broström Repair With and Without Augmentation Using Suture Tape for Chronic Lateral Ankle Instability. Orthop Surg 2019;11(4):671–8.

37. Stetson W, Ferkel RD. Ankle Arthroscopy: II. Indications and Results. J Am Acad Orthop Surg 1996;4(1):24–34.

38. Komenda GA, Ferkel RD. Arthroscopic findings associated with the unstable ankle. Foot Ankle Int 1999;20(11):708–13.

39. Staats K, Sabeti-Aschraf M, Apprich S, et al. Preoperative MRI is helpful but not sufficient to detect associated lesions in patients with chronic ankle instability. Knee Surg Sports Traumatol Arthrosc 2018;26(7):2103–9.

40. Berlet GC, Saar WE, Ryan A, et al. Thermal-assisted capsular modification for functional ankle instability. Foot Ankle Clin 2002;7(3):567–76, ix.

41. de Vries JS, Krips R, Blankevoort L, et al. Arthroscopic capsular shrinkage for chronic ankle instability with thermal radiofrequency: prospective multicenter trial. Orthopedics 2008;31(7):655.
42. Maiotti M, Massoni C, Tarantino U. The use of arthroscopic thermal shrinkage to treat chronic lateral ankle instability in young athletes. Arthroscopy 2005;21(6): 751–7.
43. Hawkins RB. Arthroscopic stapling repair for chronic lateral instability. Clin Podiatr Med Surg 1987;4(4):875–83.
44. Ferkel RD, Scranton PE. Arthroscopy of the ankle and foot. J Bone Joint Surg Am 1993;75(8):1233–42.
45. Acevedo JI, Mangone P. Arthroscopic Brostrom Technique. Foot Ankle Int 2015; 36(4):465–73.
46. Brown AJ, Shimozono Y, Hurley ET, et al. Arthroscopic Repair of Lateral Ankle Ligament for Chronic Lateral Ankle Instability: A Systematic Review. Arthroscopy 2018;34(8):2497–503.
47. Matsui K, Burgesson B, Takao M, et al. Minimally invasive surgical treatment for chronic ankle instability: a systematic review. Knee Surg Sports Traumatol Arthrosc 2016;24(4):1040–8.
48. Yeo ED, Lee K-T, Sung I-H, et al. Comparison of all-inside arthroscopic and open techniques for the modified broström procedure for ankle instability. Foot Ankle Int 2016;37(10):1037–45.
49. Lopes R, Andrieu M, Cordier G, et al. Arthroscopic treatment of chronic ankle instability: Prospective study of outcomes in 286 patients. Orthop Traumatol Surg Res 2018;104(8S):S199–205.

Peroneal Tendinosis and Subluxation

Julian G. Lugo-Pico, MD[a], Joshua T. Kaiser, BS[b], Rafael A. Sanchez, MD[a], Amiethab A. Aiyer, MD[c],*

KEYWORDS

- Peroneal tendons • Tendinosis • Tenosynovitis • Subluxation • Treatment
- Rehabilitation

KEY POINTS

- Peroneal tendinosis and peroneal subluxation are uncommon but lifestyle-limiting conditions that worsen if not properly diagnosed and treated.
- Adequate knowledge of the ankle anatomy, along with a detailed history and comprehensive physical examination, is essential to accurately diagnose such pathology.
- Conservative management remains first-line treatment of these injuries, but surgery is indicated if there is a failure to improve with conservative measures.
- Surgical technique varies depending on the type, mechanism, and severity of injury, but most procedures have a high success rate, with a short average return to full athletic activity.

INTRODUCTION

The lateral compartment of the leg contains the peroneal longus and brevis muscles, the primary pronators and evertors of the foot and ankle. These tendons are repetitively subjected to large weight-bearing loads that can lead to overuse injuries. Serving also as dynamic stabilizers to the lateral ankle, these tendons are also at risk during ankle inversion injuries. Peroneal tendinopathy can manifest broadly, as peroneal tendinosis, tenosynovitis, degenerative or acute ruptures, and peroneal tendon subluxation or dislocation. Accurate diagnosis of these injuries is accomplished with a detailed history and clinical examination, supplemented by imaging modalities. In the athlete, therapeutic options vary by diagnosis, and are dictated based on clinical findings. Both conservative and surgical management are appropriate.

[a] Orthopaedic Surgery, University of Miami, Jackson Memorial Hospital, 1611 Northwest 12th Avenue, Miami, FL 33136, USA; [b] University of Miami Miller School of Medicine, 1600 Northwest 10th Avenue, Miami, FL 33136, USA; [c] Foot & Ankle Service, Department of Orthopaedics, University of Miami Miller School of Medicine, 1611 Northwest 12th Avenue, Miami, FL 33136, USA
* Corresponding author.
E-mail address: Tabsaiyer@gmail.com

Clin Sports Med 39 (2020) 845–858
https://doi.org/10.1016/j.csm.2020.07.005
0278-5919/20/© 2020 Elsevier Inc. All rights reserved.
sportsmed.theclinics.com

ANATOMY AND PHYSIOLOGY

The peroneus longus and peroneus brevis are two of the muscles in the lateral compartment of the leg. Their tendons track from the distal leg, coursing posterior to the lateral ankle before inserting in the midfoot and metatarsals. Together, they evert and pronate the foot, and also function as secondary ankle plantarflexors.[1] Knowledge of the lateral ankle and peroneal tendon anatomy and biomechanics is vital in identifying factors that contribute to peroneal tendon pathology.

The peroneus longus originates from the anterolateral proximal two-thirds of the fibula, and the fascia of the anterior and posterior intermuscular septum of the leg. Its tendon passes around the lateral aspect of the cuboid, courses through the plantar midfoot, then inserts at the plantar lateral margin of the base of the first metatarsal and the medial cuneiform. The peroneus brevis originates from the distal two-thirds of the anterolateral fibula and the intermuscular septum, and its tendon inserts distally onto the styloid process of the fifth metatarsal base.[1,2]

Together, these tendons traverse the posterior aspect of the distal fibula inside a common synovial sheath that originates approximately 2.5 to 3.5 cm proximal to the tip of the fibula. Whereas the longus muscle becomes tendinous approximately 2 to 3 cm proximal to the ankle, the brevis muscle retains muscle fibers until the level of the ankle.[3] The peroneus brevis is located directly posterior on the fibula, whereas the peroneus longus is located posterolaterally to the brevis tendon. The pair courses within the retromalleolar groove to the tip of the distal fibula.[1] The architecture of this groove is variable between patients, in depth and morphology. In approximately 80% of cases, the retromalleolar groove is concave, but about 20% of patients present with a shallow, convex, or even absent groove. It is proposed that this subset of patients may be at increased risk of tendon subluxation or dislocation.[2,4] The sulcus is typically accompanied by a fibrocartilaginous ridge extending off the posterolateral border of the fibula, which acts to increase the depth of the groove and prevent such pathology.[1]

Distal to the fibular tip, the tendons course above (brevis) or below (longus) the peroneal tubercle on the lateral surface of the calcaneus. The tendons lie superficial to the calcaneofibular ligament and deep to the superior peroneal retinaculum (SPR), a stabilizing band of fascia extending from the posterolateral surface of the fibula to the lateral calcaneus and Achilles tendon sheath.[1,5] Both the calcaneofibular ligament and the SPR help stabilize the peroneal tendons at the distal edge of the retromalleolar sulcus. They are especially vital in preventing subluxation during the gait cycle.

There is a bifurcation of the common synovial sheath at the inferior margin of the SPR. The tendons then travel separately as they course toward the calcaneal peroneal tubercle.[6] At the level of the tubercle, the tendons are further restrained by the inferior peroneal retinaculum. The peroneus brevis passes dorsal to the tubercle before coursing distally toward its insertion site at the base of the fifth metatarsal. The peroneus longus courses plantar/inferior to the tubercle, and turns medially around cuboid notch to course along the plantar aspect of the foot. The tendon then progresses obliquely across the plantar surface, ultimately inserting on the medial cuneiform and base of the first metatarsal.[1,2,4] While passing anteromedially across the plantar midfoot (the plantar peroneal tunnel), the longus tendon is covered by a synovial sheath.[1]

It may be beneficial to organize peroneal anatomy and the related pathology by dividing the area into four zones. Brandes and Smith initially introduced this concept, and it was later modified by Sammarco.[7,8] Zone A is bounded by the distal fibula and the SPR. Zone B focuses on the inferior peroneal retinaculum at the level of the peroneal tubercle. Zone C highlights the osseous depression in the lateral cuboid, where the peroneus longus begins its plantar course. Zone D is most distal and covers the plantar surface.[8]

The peroneal tendons are located lateral to the subtalar joint and produce most of the hindfoot eversion power.[2] The peroneus brevis is also the main abductor of the midfoot and hindfoot, whereas the peroneus longus plantarflexes the first metatarsal. The os peroneum, a fibrocartilaginous sesamoid bone, can sometimes be seen within the peroneus longus tendon at the point where the longus tendon courses the cuboid notch. The os peroneum provides mechanical advantage for ankle plantarflexion.[1] Both peroneal muscles are important active stabilizers against inversion-supination sprains, and the peroneus longus also helps stabilize the ankle during passive inversion-supination.[2,9] The muscles are innervated at their proximal end by the superficial peroneal nerve. Distally, superficial branches of the sural nerve course over the tendons but provide no additional motor innervation.[5] Both tendons are supplied by the posterior peroneal artery (**Fig. 1**).[2,10]

PATHOPHYSIOLOGY AND COMMON MECHANISMS OF INJURY

The incidence of peroneal tendon injuries is unknown but is likely underreported in the literature secondary to missed or misdiagnosis of peroneal pathology.[7] In a study of 40 patients who underwent surgical repair of peroneal tendon pathology, only 60% of subjects were correctly diagnosed on initial evaluation.[11] Furthermore, peroneal tenosynovitis was identified in 77% of patients undergoing lateral ligament ankle reconstruction for chronic instability.[12]

The most common manifestation of acute injuries occurs during inversion ankle sprains. At 15° to 25° plantarflexion, the tendons are under eccentric load tension, causing them to perch along the distal anterolateral fibula, thereby increasing their vulnerability to injury during ankle inversion.[2] Recurrent ankle sprains, in addition to other mechanisms, such as chronic overuse or repeated minor trauma, can also contribute to peroneal tendon injuries. Injuries may manifest as tendonitis, tenosynovitis, rupture, or chronic subluxation/dislocation.[2,13]

Peroneal Tendinosis/Stenosing Tenosynovitis

Peroneal tendinosis typically results from aggregated microtrauma caused by a wide range of peroneal pathology but may also be a concomitant result of acute ankle trauma.[2,14] Endurance runners, ballet dancers, and basketball and soccer players have frequently been identified in overuse injury.[2,4,14] Poorly fitting footwear,

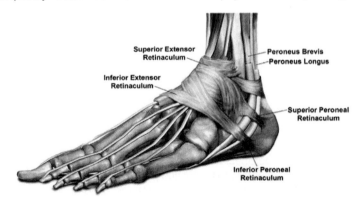

Fig. 1. Schematic illustration of the peroneal complex, highlighting the peroneus brevis, peroneus longus, SPR, and inferior peroneal retinaculum. (*From* Kumar Y, Alian A, Ahlawat S, et al. Peroneal tendon pathology: Pre- and post-operative high resolution US and MR imaging. Eur J Radiol. 2017;92:132-144; with permission.)

particularly ski boots and hockey skates, may also aggravate the tendons, causing inflammation, hypertrophy, and eventual scarring.[14]

A host of variations in ankle anatomy have been implicated as risk factors of tendinosis, with enlarged peroneal tubercle, low-lying peroneus brevis muscle at the level of the tubercle, and/or presence of a peroneus quartus or peroneal quintus muscle being the most common causes.[2,15,16] Subfibular impingement in the setting of pes planovalgus alignment or secondary to calcaneal malunion has also been identified.[17] Meanwhile, the peroneus brevis is at increased risk for tendinopathy because of an increased risk for entrapment against the fibula or calcaneus by the peroneus longus.[14]

Stenosing tenosynovitis is a unique manifestation of ankle trauma and overuse. Lateral wall blowout after intra-articular calcaneal fracture, inversion ankle sprains, abnormal anatomy of the retromalleolar sulcus and lateral calcaneal tubercle, and peroneal tubercle osteochondroma have all been identified as predisposing risk factors for tenosynovitis. Cavovarus foot alignment has also been implicated.[18] The inflammation most often occurs in the common synovial sheath, but also may occur more distally in either individual tendon sheath. Tenosynovitis involving solely the peroneus longus is often a related finding in painful os peroneum syndrome, and patients present with tendon and sheath calcification.[1,14] Coexistence of peroneal tenosynovitis in patients undergoing surgery for correction of peroneal subluxation is well documented in previous literature, especially in cases where lateral ankle instability was also present.[4,12,19]

Peroneal Subluxation/Dislocation

Peroneal dislocation and recurrent subluxation typically manifest as a result of injury to the SPR, the primary ligamentous restraint of the tendons in the distal ankle. Other risk factors include a shallow or convex retromalleolar groove and lateral ankle instability.[1] The most common injury mechanism involves forceful contraction of the peroneals during sudden dorsiflexion from stopping or landing while the ankle is in a nonneutral position.[20] The force generated by the taut tendons overcomes the restraint provided by the SPR and the fibrocartilage ridge at the distal retromalleolar sulcus.[1,2]

Intrasheath subluxation has also been identified in the literature but has not been extensively studied. Type A involves the subluxation of intact peroneal tendons over each other while remaining within an intact SPR. Type B involves the subluxation of the longus tendon through a longitudinally split brevis tendon.[21,22]

The exact mechanism of subluxation cannot be discretely identified because the injury pattern has been identified in multiple varieties of sprains and in direct trauma.[14] Patients who have sustained acute tendon dislocation may also present with additional injury to the ankle. Such comorbidities include calcaneus and talus fractures, Achilles tendon rupture, and ligament sprains.[1,2,6]

CLINICAL EVALUATION AND DIAGNOSIS
History and Physical Examination

Although the incidence of peroneal tendinosis, dislocation, or subluxation is low, it is important to consider in patients with lateral and posterolateral ankle pain. Because of potential involvement in acute and chronic injury patterns, a thorough history is essential in the diagnosis of peroneal pathology. Complaints associated with peroneal pathology include lateral hindfoot pain, swelling, and/or weakness, and episodes of ankle instability, or "giving way," while walking or during exercise.[14] As such, pertinent comorbidities should be explored; this includes inquiries about previous ankle sprains or fractures, and a dedicated examination of ligamentous integrity.[2,20] Past medical history must rule out other potential causes for similar presentations, such as rheumatoid or psoriatic arthritis, hyperparathyroidism, and peripheral neuropathy.[23] Previous treatment and treatment response should also be explored.

Inspection and palpation of the tendons is an important part of the foot and ankle examination. Inflammation and associated swelling of the tendons may be noticeable on examination. Palpation along the course of the peroneals should be performed at rest and during active contraction. Warmth and tenderness may be indicative of acute or acute-on-chronic inflammation.[2] Hindfoot alignment should also be assessed because varus alignment is a risk factor for peroneal tendon pathology.[23] In cases of tendon overuse and entrapment, synovial hypertrophy and repetitive tendon microtrauma can produce excessive stress on the tendons, which may contribute to calcifications.[14] Passive hindfoot inversion and plantarflexion and actively resisted hindfoot eversion and ankle dorsiflexion may exacerbate symptoms of pain or weakness. Dorsiflexion and inversion can also elicit evidence of peroneal subluxation.[1,14,23]

Popularized by Sobel and colleagues, the peroneal tunnel compression test is used to evaluate for peroneal brevis tendonitis and SPR integrity. The test is accomplished by palpating the fibular groove and SPR while having the patient evert and dorsiflex the foot and ankle against resistance. A positive test elicits snapping, popping, or subluxation of the tendons with concurrent pain.[24]

Peroneal dislocation most often occurs during athletic competition, particularly skiing, ice skating, soccer, basketball, rugby, and gymnastics.[1] Patients complain of nonspecific pain and swelling with characteristic visible tendon snapping or popping.[1,23] Persistent, isolated dislocation is not common in the acute setting; however, chronic subluxation may also be confused with ankle instability, although the two entities can both be present in many cases. Subluxation can also be reproduced by isolating and rotating the ankle while stabilizing the lower leg.[23] The tendons may remain "locked" outside the distal edge of the fibula, requiring manual reduction.[1]

Imaging

Initial imaging of foot and ankle injuries should always begin with the conventional weightbearing radiographs. Plain radiographs provide an initial overview of the bony anatomy, confirm or exclude potential diagnoses, and help determine a potential need for advanced imaging.[25] Despite its limitations, standard three-view, weightbearing radiography is useful in the evaluation of peroneal pathology. Radiographs can highlight avulsion of the lateral malleolus or avulsion of the insertion of the SPR, a common finding in traumatic peroneal dislocation injuries.[2,6] Such injury is best visualized on an internal rotation (mortise) view of the ankle joint.[4,20] Likewise, peroneal tubercle hypertrophy, a potential cause of tendinopathy, is adequately identified on radiograph.[20] Hindfoot alignment radiographs are also obtained to better assess any deformity that could predispose a patient to peroneal injuries.

Computerized tomography scans confer some value in peroneal pathology and are best used to define bony abnormalities and potential occult fractures. Peroneal tubercle enlargement and lateral malleolus avulsions are readily identified with this modality (**Fig. 2**).[23]

Ultrasonography may also be useful. Ultrasound displays high spatial resolution and provides the advantage of real-time analysis, which is particularly important in the identification of tendon subluxation. Dynamic ultrasonography displayed a 100% positive predictive value in 12 patients with suspected subluxation, confirmed by findings during surgery.[26] Ultrasound can also be useful to assess for fluid collection greater

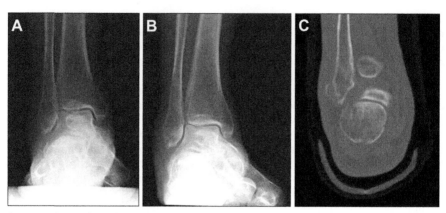

Fig. 2. Radiograph and computed tomography imaging of an SPR avulsion. (*A, B*) Non-weightbearing radiographs show the fleck sign of the distal malleolus, consistent with an SPR avulsion. (*C*) Axial computed tomography image of the distal fibula indicating lateral malleolar avulsion.

than 1 mm and/or tendon hypertrophy, two findings indicative of peroneal tendinosis.[20,23] Tendinosis presents as hypoechoic swelling, whereas tenosynovitis is visualized with tendon thickening, an anechoic area surrounding the tendon that is indicative of synovial effusion, and a hypoechoic synovial sheath.[27]

MRI remains the most detailed modality for visualization of the peroneal tendons, capable of evaluating for peroneal tendonitis, tenosynovitis, and SPR integrity. Images should be captured with the ankle in 20° plantarflexion. Such positioning limits the magic angle effect of MRI, a phenomenon of artifactual hyperintensity caused by tendons or collagenous structures positioned at a 55° angle with the main magnetic vector. Because of the abrupt change of course of the tendons at the ankle, such hyperintensity can falsely indicate the presence of peroneal tendinopathy. The magic angle effect is more likely to influence sequences with a short echo time, such as T1-weighted images.[28] As such, STIR and T2-weighted fat-suppressed sequences should be used.[29]

Axial MRIs provide the best visualization of the entirety of the complex and related bony anatomy, whereas sagittal images are used to assess the extent of tendon disease.[28] Tendons without injury display homogenous low intensity on T1- and T2-weighted and STIR imaging. Tenosynovitis, tendinosis, and other cases of tendon disease display heterogeneity and increased signal intensity on all images because of tendon thickening, tendon injury, or fluid accumulation.[20,28] However, a small area of increased intensity from the tendons within their sheath is not uncommon on T2-weighted and STIR imaging.[2]

Careful study of the SPR on MRI is important to assess for anatomic defects that are contributing to peroneal subluxation. SPR injuries were first classified by Eckert and Davis and later revised by Oden.[20] Grade I injuries are most common (51% of cases), and are classified by retinaculum attachment to the periosteum, but with periosteal elevation of the lateral malleolus by the tendons, creating a pouch into which the tendons can subluxate.[1] In grade II lesions, the SPR is separated posteriorly from the malleolus and the periosteum, with additional fibrocartilaginous ridge elevation. Grade III lesions are the second most common presentation and involve separation of the SPR from the periosteum, with the presence of fibular avulsion.[20,27,30,31] Grade IV was added by Oden to include SPR separation from its posterior attachments to the calcaneus and the deep investing fascia of the Achilles tendon. The retinaculum is found lying deep to the tendons, between the tendons and retromalleolar sulcus, thus prohibiting tendinous relocation (**Fig. 3**).[20,31]

TREATMENT OPTIONS
Conservative Treatment

Initial treatment of peroneal tendinosis is nonoperative. Early diagnosis and immediate treatment of peroneal tendon sheath disorders may help prevent progression to more complex injuries, such as tendon rupture.[32] Treatment is dictated by symptoms and includes modalities, such as nonsteroidal anti-inflammatory drugs, ice/heat therapy, and bracing, with or without formal physical therapy. Steroid or nonsteroidal anti-inflammatory drug injection directly into the tendon sheath may also be used for diagnostic and therapeutic purposes but should be used with caution, because it could be associated with increased rate of tendon rupture.[2,20] During exercise or activity, ankle braces and lateral wedge orthotics can be used to unload the peroneals to prevent additional injury.

Alternatively, 3- to 6-week periods of immobilization with a controlled ankle motion boot may be an effective treatment option in cases with severe tendinosis symptoms.[2,20] Immobilization maintains secure reduction of the tendons within the retromalleolar groove, which may maximize healing and limit scar tissue formation.[1] However, the response rate to conservative immobilization varies widely based on peroneal pathology. Immobilization is generally effective in treating tendinopathy.[33] However, immobilization is not nearly as efficacious in treating peroneal dislocation. Patients should be warned of a 50% chance of recurrent dislocation even after immobilization. Thus, such treatment is cautiously offered to nonathletes and is not recommended for high-level athletes.[16] Furthermore, prolonged immobilization demonstrates no benefit to patients with chronic subluxation, regardless of activity level.[20,30,34] Physical therapy to optimize proprioception, neuromuscular training, and peroneal tendon activation/strengthening should be initiated once the patient's pain and swelling has improved. In cases of subluxation, physical therapy may not be beneficial, especially if strengthening exercises lead to recurrent episodes of subluxation.[20]

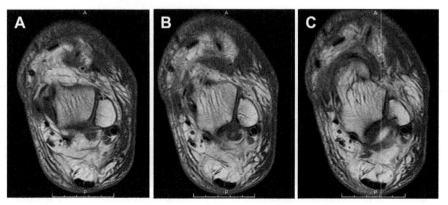

Fig. 3. MRI of peroneal tendon dislocation. (A–C). Axial MRI sections, highlighting lateral dislocation of the peroneal tendons out of the retromalleolar groove.

Surgical Treatment: Peroneal Tendinopathy (Tendinosis/Tenosynovitis)

Surgical intervention may be indicated for tendinopathy if symptoms persist despite exhausting nonsurgical alternatives. Goals of surgery include treatment of the peroneal injury and correction of any underlying causes that may be predisposing to the pathology. Such factors include ligamentous instability, varus hindfoot, or anatomic abnormalities previously discussed.[2,16,20]

Open debridement and synovectomy of the peroneal tendons remains common for the correction of tendinopathy. The tendon sheath is identified and incised to allow for direct inspection of the tendon. Diseased areas and significant tears are debrided if they involve less than 50% of the tendon cross-sectional area.[2,20] The tendon may be tubularized under direct visualization. The tendons are evaluated while the ankle is passively ranged through its full range of motion, and any subluxation or dislocation is noted. If the tendons maintain their position within the retromalleolar sulcus, the retinaculum is repaired, and the skin is approximated in layers (**Fig. 4**).[2]

For the athlete focused on returning to previous level of activity, endoscopic tendoscopy has become a popular option for the management of tendinosis or tenosynovitis. Endoscopic evaluation of the peroneal tendons confers advantages to open synovectomy because it is more focused on preserving anatomy and can also be performed under regional or local anesthetic to allow for dynamic evaluation.[35] In cases of tendoscopy, the peroneal tendons are divided into three anatomic zones, from proximal to distal.[32] Zone 1 includes common peroneal sheath and its contents, from the musculocutaneous junction to the peroneal tubercle. Zone 2 begins at peroneal tubercle and SPR, at the separation of the tendon sheaths. Zone 3 includes only the peroneus longus along on the sole.[32]

In tendoscopy, two main portal entries are made superficial to the tendons, with one port 1.5 to 2 cm distal to the posterior edge of the lateral malleolus and the second port 2 to 2.5 cm proximal to the same landmark.[35] A third, middle incision is sometimes

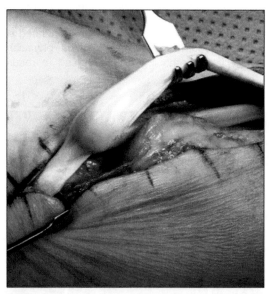

Fig. 4. Stenosis and proximal enlargement of the peroneal brevis at the level of the inferior peroneal retinaculum. (*From* Roster B, Michelier P, Giza E. Peroneal Tendon Disorders. *Clin Sports Med.* 2015;34(4):6225-641; with permission.)

required directly at the posterior edge of the lateral malleolus. Visualization of the tendon sheaths is primarily accomplished with a 30° 2.7-mm arthroscope, which is preferred to a 4-mm scope because it is easier to insert within the sheath, despite its more limited visual field. Saline injections within the sheath can often facilitate access to the tendons and enhance visualization.[2,8]

Even more recently, needle or "nano" arthroscopy has been developed, which allows for dynamic, office-based evaluation.[36,37] Procedures are completed under local anesthesia with a one-time-use, camera-tipped scope that is typically smaller than 2 mm in diameter. The procedure is indicated for a range of intra-articular pathology. It may become a more popular option in the future because the procedure is time-sensitive and allows for real-time patient feedback. Outcome data are limited but have been positive to date, with a risk profile similar to that of office-based ankle injections.[36,37]

Surgical Treatment: Peroneal Subluxation/Dislocation

Treatment protocol of peroneal subluxation remains mildly controversial for the greater population, but surgery is generally recommended as first-line treatment of athletes because of risk of long-term sequelae, such as recurrent dislocation, peroneal tendon rupture or degeneration, chronic lateral ankle pain, and tendonitis.[14,16,18]

In the athlete, the primary goals of surgery are to repair the SPR and deepen the retromalleolar sulcus if needed.[16] Additionally, any retinacular avulsions, fibular fractures, or gross anatomic abnormalities must also be addressed.[2,14,38] Many surgical techniques have been described to achieve this goal. Such procedures include retromalleolar groove deepening with either tissue transfers to reconstruct the SPR or bone block procedures to improve the functional anatomy of the fibular fibrocartilaginous rim.[2,20] Excision of low-lying peroneus brevis muscle belly and reconstruction of the SPR using drill holes in the posterior aspect of the fibula has yielded excellent results. Care should be taken to ensure that the SPR is imbricated and attached securely to prevent recurrent subluxation. Superior retinaculoplasty for grade I and II injuries without any additional pathology may also be performed endoscopically, conferring the same benefits typically afforded by minimally invasive surgery, such as improved acute postoperative results and shorter return to full activity (**Figs. 5** and **6**).[39,40]

POSTOPERATIVE PROTOCOL AND OUTCOMES

Following surgery, the ankle is temporarily immobilized to allow for healing of the surgical incision and resolution of postoperative swelling. Surgeon preference and intraoperative findings usually dictate the type of immobilization used. In debridement and synovectomy cases, a soft dressing may be applied acutely, followed by a removable brace that allows some degree of early mobilization to prevent scar tissue formation.[41,42] Early mobilization of the tendons with active range of motion exercises is encouraged, especially in the athletic population, to promote accelerated rehabilitation and minimize adhesions and scarring development.[43,44] However, in cases where the SPR has been repaired and/or bony work has been performed, the ankle is typically immobilized with a controlled ankle motion boot anywhere from 2 to 6 weeks, with a minimum of 2 weeks nonweightbearing.[16,45] Casting may lead to excessive stiffness and difficulty with tendon excursion, especially in the athletic population where accelerated rehabilitation timelines are preferred.[46]

The patient can progress to full weightbearing and physical therapy as tolerated but should refrain from resisted eversion maneuvers until at least 4 weeks postoperatively.[2,46] Therapy should include phased muscle firing and joint mobilization initially,

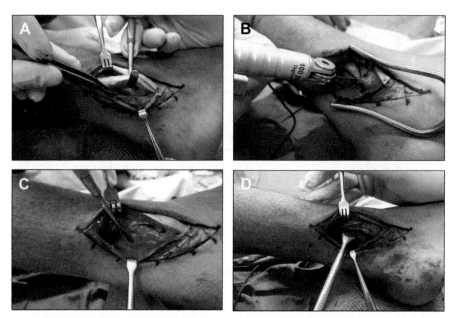

Fig. 5. Retromalleolar groove deepening procedure. (*A*) The peroneal tendons are exposed and later retracted for protection purposes. (*B*) The retromalleolar sulcus is explored before osteotomy. (*C*) Osteotomy is performed to increase the depth of the retromalleolar sulcus. (*D*) The cancellous bone is tamped to manually increase sulcus depth.

followed by balance and proprioception training, and lastly dynamic strength exercises that allow a return to full activity.[20,41]

Surgical outcomes for peroneal tendinosis generally are positive, but have not been reported extensively in the athlete population. A 19-patient cohort who underwent synovectomy to correct tenosynovitis reported encouraging outcomes, with 16 patients symptom free at the end of 8 weeks.[19] Furthermore, Kennedy and colleagues[41] identified 23 cases of peroneal tendoscopy, focusing on functional outcomes. All but two patients reported significant improvement compared with baseline using the foot and ankle outcome score with little to no complications. A study involving 17 patients who underwent surgery to correct tendinopathy in the absence of subluxation had an average return to sport of 8.5 months. Although the range of return to sport outcomes was dramatic, from 3 months to 3 years, 16 of 17 patients reported satisfaction with the procedure.[47]

Patients undergoing surgical management of peroneal subluxation have also demonstrated positive results. A study of 55 outcomes for SPR repair in the setting of recurrent peroneal subluxation demonstrated 100% return to full activity, with an average time to full clearance for activity of 3 months.[48] Other studies indicate similar outcomes. Saxena and Ewen[48] reported that a cohort of 31 athletic patients who underwent surgery for SPR reconstruction with additional peroneal tendon repair demonstrated 100% return to sport with an average time of 3.2 months until full clearance. Additionally, Porter and colleagues[46] performed groove deepening and concurrent SPR reconstruction on 14 athletes, with an average return to full activity of 3 months and no recurrent subluxation at 35 months follow-up, despite implementing an accelerated rehabilitation program.

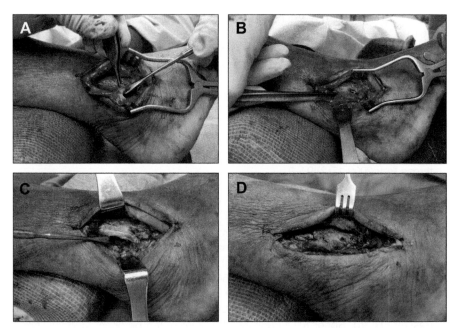

Fig. 6. SPR repair with fibular groove deepening. (*A*) The peroneal tendons are retracted, exposing the attenuated SPR, adjacent to the forceps. (*B, C*) Before SPR repair, the fibular retromalleolar groove is deepened to improve osseous stability. (*D*) The SPR is fully repaired following groove deepening.

SUMMARY

Although uncommon, peroneal tendinosis and peroneal subluxation and dislocation are potentially lifestyle-limiting conditions that can worsen if not properly diagnosed and treated. Adequate knowledge of the ankle anatomy, along with a detailed history and comprehensive physical examination, is essential to accurately diagnose such pathology. Imagining modalities, such as radiograph, MRI, and ultrasound, are useful in the diagnosis of peroneal tendinopathy. Conservative measures remain as the first line of treatment, but surgery is often indicated in cases that fail to improve. Depending on the type, mechanism, and severity of the injury, various surgical techniques are used, many with a high rate of success, minimal complications, and a short return to unrestricted activity.

DISCLOSURE

The authors have no commercial or financial conflicts of interest to disclose.

REFERENCES

1. Jeng C. Peroneal tendon disorders. In: Altchek DW, DiGiovanni CW, Dines JS, et al, editors. Foot and ankle sports medicine. Philadelphia: Wolters Kluwer; 2013. p. 141–9.
2. Roster B, Michelier P, Giza E. Peroneal tendon disorders. Clin Sports Med 2015; 34(4):625–41.
3. Baxter DE, Porter DA, Schon L. Baxter's the foot and ankle in sport. 2nd edition. Philadelphia: Mosby Elsevier; 2008.

4. Berquist TH. Imaging of the foot and ankle. Philadelphia: Wolters Kluwer Health; 2010.

5. Patel A, Horton G. Anatomy of the foot and ankle. In: Altchek DW, DiGiovanni CW, Dines JS, et al, editors. Foot and ankle sports medicine. Philadelphia: Wolters Kluwer; 2012. p. 1–10.

6. Brage ME, Hansen ST Jr. Traumatic subluxation/dislocation of the peroneal tendons. Foot Ankle 1992;13(7):423–31.

7. Brandes CB, Smith RW. Characterization of patients with primary peroneus longus tendinopathy: a review of twenty-two cases. Foot Ankle Int 2000;21(6):462–8.

8. Sammarco VJ. Peroneal tendoscopy: indications and techniques. Sports Med Arthrosc Rev 2009;17(2):94–9.

9. Ziai P, Benca E, von Skrbensky G, et al. The role of the peroneal tendons in passive stabilisation of the ankle joint: an in vitro study. Knee Surg Sports Traumatol Arthrosc 2013;21(6):1404–8.

10. Kumar Y, Alian A, Ahlawat S, et al. Peroneal tendon pathology: pre- and postoperative high resolution US and MR imaging. Eur J Radiol 2017;92:132–44.

11. Dombek MF, Lamm BM, Saltrick K, et al. Peroneal tendon tears: a retrospective review. J Foot Ankle Surg 2003;42(5):250–8.

12. Digiovanni BF, Fraga CJ, Cohen BE, et al. Associated injuries found in chronic lateral ankle instability. Foot Ankle Int 2000;21(10):809–15.

13. Bassett FH 3rd, Speer KP. Longitudinal rupture of the peroneal tendons. Am J Sports Med 1993;21(3):354–7.

14. Sammarco VJ, Sammarco GJ. Injuries to the tibialis anterior, peroneal tendons, and long flexors of the toes. In: Baxter DE, Porter DA, Schon L, editors. Baxter's the foot and ankle in sport. 2nd edition. Philadelphia: Mosby Elsevier; 2008. p. 121–46.

15. Hyer CF, Dawson JM, Philbin TM, et al. The peroneal tubercle: description, classification, and relevance to peroneus longus tendon pathology. Foot Ankle Int 2005;26(11):947–50.

16. van Dijk PA, Miller D, Calder J, et al. The ESSKA-AFAS international consensus statement on peroneal tendon pathologies. Knee Surg Sports Traumatol Arthrosc 2018;26(10):3096–107.

17. Kaplan RMJ, Aiyer MA, Nguyen TD, et al. Subfibular impingement: current concepts, imaging findings and management strategies. Curr Orthop Pract 2019; 30(1):69–76.

18. Padanilam T. Disorders of the anterior tibial, peroneal, and Achilles tendons. In: Chou LB, editor. Orthopaedic knowledge update. Foot and ankle 5. Rosemont (IL): American Academy of Orthopaedic Surgeons; 2014.

19. Gray JM, Alpar EK. Peroneal tenosynovitis following ankle sprains. Injury 2001; 32(6):487–9.

20. Philbin TM, Landis GS, Smith B. Peroneal tendon injuries. J Am Acad Orthop Surg 2009;17(5):306–17.

21. Guelfi M, Vega J, Malagelada F, et al. Tendoscopic treatment of peroneal intrasheath subluxation: a new subgroup with superior peroneal retinaculum injury. Foot Ankle Int 2018;39(5):542–50.

22. Raikin SM, Elias I, Nazarian LN. Intrasheath subluxation of the peroneal tendons. J Bone Joint Surg Am 2008;90(5):992–9.

23. Selmani E, Gjata V, Gjika E. Current concepts review: peroneal tendon disorders. Foot Ankle Int 2006;27(3):221–8.

24. Sobel M, Geppert MJ, Olson EJ, et al. The dynamics of peroneus brevis tendon splits: a proposed mechanism, technique of diagnosis, and classification of injury. Foot Ankle 1992;13(7):413–22.

25. Pavlov H, Sofka CM, Saboeiro GR, et al. Imaging of foot and ankle athletic injuries. In: Altchek DW, DiGiovanni CW, Dines JS, et al, editors. Foot and ankle sports medicine. Philadelphia: Wolters Kluwer; 2012. p. 51–66.

26. Neustadter J, Raikin SM, Nazarian LN. Dynamic sonographic evaluation of peroneal tendon subluxation. AJR Am J Roentgenol 2004;183(4):985–8.

27. Lee SJ, Jacobson JA, Kim SM, et al. Ultrasound and MRI of the peroneal tendons and associated pathology. Skeletal Radiol 2013;42(9):1191–200.

28. Wang XT, Rosenberg ZS, Mechlin MB, et al. Normal variants and diseases of the peroneal tendons and superior peroneal retinaculum: MR imaging features. Radiographics 2005;25(3):587–602.

29. Ieong E, Rafferty M, Khanna M, et al. Use of fat-suppressed t2-weighted MRI images to reduce the magic angle effect in peroneal tendons. Foot Ankle Spec 2018;12(6):513–7.

30. Eckert WR, Davis EA Jr. Acute rupture of the peroneal retinaculum. J Bone Joint Surg Am 1976;58(5):670–2.

31. Oden RR. Tendon injuries about the ankle resulting from skiing. Clin Orthop Relat Res 1987;(216):63–9.

32. Lui TH. Endoscopic synovectomy of peroneal tendon sheath. Arthrosc Tech 2017; 6(3):e887–92.

33. Heckman DS, Gluck GS, Parekh SG. Tendon disorders of the foot and ankle, part 1: peroneal tendon disorders. Am J Sports Med 2009;37(3):614–25.

34. Stover CN, Bryan DR. Traumatic dislocation of the peroneal tendons. Am J Surg 1962;103:180–6.

35. van Dijk C, Kort N. Tendoscopy of the peroneal tendons. Arthroscopy 1998;14(5): 471–8.

36. Labib AS, Slone SH. Office-based needle arthroscopy for the foot and ankle. Tech Foot Ankle Surg 2015;14(1):9–11.

37. Harris A. NYU Langone conducts first foot & ankle arthroscopic treatment with new visualization technology [press release]. New York: NYU Langone Health Office of Media Relations; September 16, 2019.

38. Irwin TA. DeLee, Drez & Miller's orthopaedic sports medicine: principles and practice. In: Miller MD, Thompson SR, Aiyer AA, et al, editors. DeLee and Drez's orthopaedic sports medicine. 5th edition. Philadelphia: Elsevier; 2019. p. 1462–83.

39. Lui TH. Endoscopic peroneal retinaculum reconstruction. Knee Surg Sports Traumatol Arthrosc 2006;14(5):478–81.

40. van Dijk PA, Gianakos AL, Kerkhoffs GM, et al. Return to sports and clinical outcomes in patients treated for peroneal tendon dislocation: a systematic review. Knee Surg Sports Traumatol Arthrosc 2016;24:1155–64.

41. Kennedy JG, van Dijk PA, Murawski CD, et al. Functional outcomes after peroneal tendoscopy in the treatment of peroneal tendon disorders. Knee Surg Sports Traumatol Arthrosc 2016;24(4):1148–54.

42. Marmotti A, Cravino M, Germano M, et al. Peroneal tendoscopy. Curr Rev Musculoskelet Med 2012;5(2):135–44.

43. van Dijk PAD, Lubberts B, Verheul C, et al. Rehabilitation after surgical treatment of peroneal tendon tears and ruptures. Knee Surg Sports Traumatol Arthrosc 2016;24(4):1165–74.

44. Urguden M, Gulten IA, Civan O, et al. Results of peroneal tendoscopy with a technical modification. Foot Ankle Int 2018;40(3):356–63.

45. Saragas NP, Ferrao PN, Mayet Z, et al. Peroneal tendon dislocation/subluxation: case series and review of the literature. Foot Ankle Surg 2016;22(2):125–30.

46. Porter D, McCarroll J, Knapp E, et al. Peroneal tendon subluxation in athletes: fibular groove deepening and retinacular reconstruction. Foot Ankle Int 2005; 26(6):436–41.

47. Grasset W, Mercier N, Chaussard C, et al. The surgical treatment of peroneal tendinopathy (excluding subluxations): a series of 17 patients. J Foot Ankle Surg 2012;51(1):13–9.

48. Saxena A, Ewen B. Peroneal subluxation: surgical results in 31 athletic patients. J Foot Ankle Surg 2010;49(3):238–41.

Painful Accessory Navicular and Spring Ligament Injuries in Athletes

John T. Campbell, MD*, Clifford L. Jeng, MD

KEYWORDS

- Accessory navicular • Spring ligament • Athletes • Calcaneonavicular • Arch pain

KEY POINTS

- Accessory navicular problems and spring ligament injuries in athletes are different entities from more common posterior tibialis tendon pathology and tears in older patients.
- Painful accessory navicular affects adolescent and young adult athletes, causing medial arch pain and weakness.
- Acute injuries of the spring ligament occur in athletes of numerous sports, often from twisting or eversion sprains.
- Diagnostic mainstays include careful physical examination, weightbearing radiographs, and MRI.
- Nonsurgical treatment can be attempted for both entities, but is often ineffective and surgery is preferred to facilitate recovery and return to play.

ACCESSORY NAVICULAR

Introduction

Accessory navicular is one of the most common accessory ossicles, with an incidence of approximately 4%.[1] It has been categorized into 3 main types[1,2] (**Fig. 1**). Type I is a small ossicle that is embedded within the distal fibers of the posterior tibialis tendon near its insertion point on the navicular tuberosity. Type II, the most common, is a larger fragment with a distinct interface or synchondrosis composed of cartilaginous or fibrous tissue adjacent to the main navicular. Type III is cornuate-shaped or partially fused to the main navicular, representing enlargement of the medial aspect of the tuberosity.

The association of an accessory navicular with a flat foot deformity has been a topic of debate. Early literature proposed that accessory naviculars lead to a pes planus deformity.[3] Kidner[3,4] felt that due to the offset position of the accessory bone, the

Institute for Foot and Ankle Reconstruction, Mercy Medical Center, 301 St. Paul Place, Baltimore, MD 21202, USA
* Corresponding author.
E-mail address: jcampbell@mdmercy.com

Clin Sports Med 39 (2020) 859–876
https://doi.org/10.1016/j.csm.2020.05.002
0278-5919/20/© 2020 Elsevier Inc. All rights reserved.

sportsmed.theclinics.com

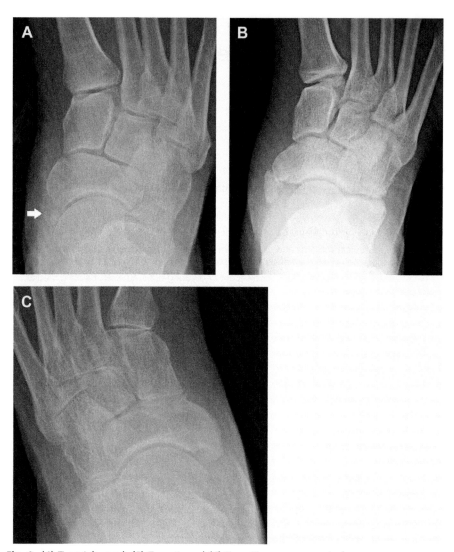

Fig. 1. (A) Type I (arrow), (B) Type II, and (C) Type III accessory naviculars.

insertion and line of pull of the posterior tibialis tendon was compromised; this resulted in mechanical disadvantage of the tendon and loss of its suspensory effect causing flattening of the arch. These concepts led to his early proposal for surgical excision and advancement of the tendon to the plantar navicular (Kidner procedure). Subsequent investigators felt there was no relation between an accessory navicular and pes planus.[5] More contemporary reports indicated that the accessory navicular can be associated with a pes planus deformity in some patients.[6] One study, for example, showed the calcaneal pitch angle in feet with an accessory navicular to be lower than controls, 14.8° versus 21°, respectively.[6] It was also noted that a Kidner procedure alone did not fully restore the height of the arch.[6] Subsequent reports have identified flatfoot incidence in patients with an accessory navicular ranging from 15% to 34%.[7–9]

Similar to pes planus due to other etiologies, contracture of the Achilles tendon or gastrocnemius muscle is often present in patients with an accessory navicular.

Clinical Evaluation

Individuals with a symptomatic accessory navicular commonly describe pain along the medial arch. In the setting of concomitant pes planus, they may also note impingement in the area of the sinus tarsi laterally. Direct pressure from the shoe or cleat on the medial side of the arch can also lead to pain.[8] Shear stress or tension in the area of the synchondrosis also produces medial arch pain.[9] Direct trauma to the area or a sprain mechanism is very common in athletes, reported in up to 35% of cases.[10] Symptoms occur during walking, running, and training activities.[8,11] It is useful to elicit a history of the previous treatments or interventions the individual has attempted, including immobilization, rest, recent changes or adjustments to the training regimen, and orthotic devices used.

Careful physical examination is essential in evaluating the athlete with a painful accessory navicular. The alignment of the foot is observed, including any valgus of the hindfoot, flattening of the medial arch, and abduction of the midfoot. Inspection of the patient's footwear may show wear of the medial portion of the sole of the athletic shoe or sneaker. The function of the posterior tibialis tendon is assessed, including manual muscle strength against resisted inversion and the ability to perform multiple single limb heel rises. Range of motion of the ankle and hindfoot is necessary to determine the degree of flexibility. The Achilles tendon is assessed by dorsiflexion of the ankle with the knee both flexed and extended; improved dorsiflexion with the knee flexed (Silfverskiold test) indicates isolated contracture of the gastrocnemius. The foot is palpated to identify areas of tenderness, including the accessory navicular, the posterior tibialis tendon from the medial malleolus to the ossicle, the medial arch, and the region of the sinus tarsi.

Standard weightbearing radiographic views of the foot are obtained including anteroposterior, lateral, and internal oblique views. An external oblique view can better characterize the size and appearance of the accessory navicular. Proximal retraction of the accessory navicular can indicate possible avulsion injury through the synchondrosis. The main body of the navicular itself is typically much wider with increased medial protrusion compared with controls.[12] Radiographs are also reviewed for the findings of pes planus, such as decreased calcaneal pitch, talonavicular uncoverage, and sag of the talo–first metatarsal angle on the lateral view (Meary angle).[7]

Additional imaging can be helpful in evaluating the painful accessory navicular. Three-phase bone scans can show increased uptake at the medial edge of the navicular, consistent with stress reaction.[1,13] Computed tomography scan is sometimes used to determine if a seeming accessory navicular is in fact an acute avulsion fragment. Rather than smooth corticated borders, an acute avulsion injury would demonstrate jagged edges consistent with an acute fracture. MRI is of particular use in evaluating these athletes and is likely the most helpful modality. MRI commonly shows edema in the accessory ossicle itself as well as the medial edge of the navicular.[8,9,14] There can be fluid or edema within the synchondrosis itself, indicating a stress reaction or possible sprain injury.[8,9] In addition, MRI can evaluate the distal aspect of the posterior tibialis tendon for any tendon damage or injury.[8,9] Ultrasound imaging of the navicular may indicate instability or hypermobility of the accessory bone.[8] Ultrasound may also show thickening or tendinosis of the posterior tibialis tendon, although this would be more prevalent in older individuals rather than the young athlete.

Nonsurgical Treatment

Initial treatment with nonoperative measures is warranted, especially in athletes.[2,9,13,15] Rest, restriction from running and training, and avoidance of activities that exacerbate symptoms are initiated. Anti-inflammatory medications and intermittent cryotherapy to the arch can assist with symptomatic relief. Orthotic insoles with medial arch posting may relieve stress on the synchondrosis and distal posterior tibialis tendon. It is often necessary to incorporate a relief underneath the accessory navicular to relieve direct pressure on it. In the presence of increased heel valgus, mild medial heel wedge posting can also be beneficial. For severe symptoms or those that are refractory to initial treatments, immobilization in a removable boot brace can be attempted. This is usually preferable to a cast, as the removable orthosis allows continued manual treatments, therapeutic exercises to work on motion and strengthening, and easier cardio training and conditioning, such as a stationary bike, antigravity treadmill, or aqua jogging.

Nonoperative treatment of a painful accessory navicular is appropriate as an initial intervention but has relatively low success rates, particularly in the athletic population.[8] One comparative series indicated nonoperative treatment was successful in only 7% of athletes versus 34% of nonathletes, indicating that athletic individuals may benefit from earlier surgical intervention.[8]

Surgical Decision Making

Patients with a painful accessory navicular who have failed appropriate nonsurgical treatment can be considered for surgical management. The team physician or treating surgeon has to carefully consider the athlete's symptom severity and ability to continue participating in the current season. In some athletes it may be possible to manage symptoms sufficiently to allow continued participation, with modified practice and treatments as detailed previously. In these cases, surgical treatment would be considered in the off-season to allow healing and rehabilitation. Surgery is considered in-season if the symptoms are particularly severe or if nonsurgical treatments and rest have proven ineffective and continued play is not possible.

The mainstay of surgical treatment for painful accessory navicular is the Kidner procedure.[3,4] Kidner popularized his surgical technique to excise the accessory bone from the medial arch[3,4,15,16] (**Fig. 2**). This was combined with plantar advancement of the posterior tibial tendon to try to reestablish better function and mechanics of the tendon.[3,4] In addition, numerous investigators have recommended trimming or shaving down the hypertrophic bone of the medial navicular, so-called naviculoplasty.[12,15–17] This is done to decrease direct pressure from the enlarged navicular, which can continue to be symptomatic even after removal of the accessory alone. Contemporary approaches to the modified Kidner procedure included use of suture anchors to reattach the posterior tibial tendon to the medial or plantar-medial edge of the navicular to allow tendon-to-cancellous bone healing[8,9,16–18] (**Fig. 3**). This has resulted in good pain relief and high satisfaction rates, including in athletes.[15,16] This may also show some improvement in arch alignment in the younger patient,[16] but most series show no improvement in arch alignment. Studies have shown improved outcome scores, including visual analogue scale (VAS) pain scores with no real difference between athletes and nonathletic individuals.[8]

Several early reports recommended simple excision of the accessory ossicle without formal advancement of the posterior tibial tendon.[2,5,13] This was felt to be a technically easier procedure and allow predictable clinical results. Several series showed similar success rates between simple excision and excision along with tendon

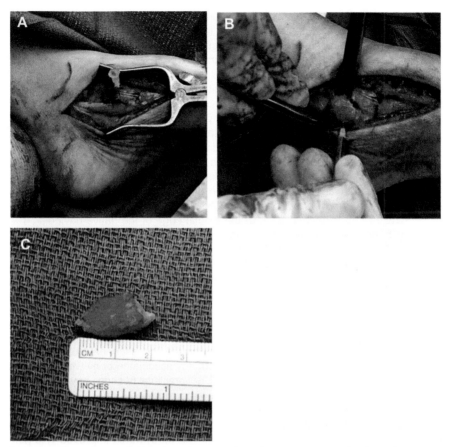

Fig. 2. (*A*) Through a medial incision, the navicular tuberosity is exposed. A hypodermic needle can be used to identify the interface between the accessory ossicle and main navicular. (*B*) The accessory bone is sharply released from the posterior tibialis tendon fibers. (*C*) Accessory navicular.

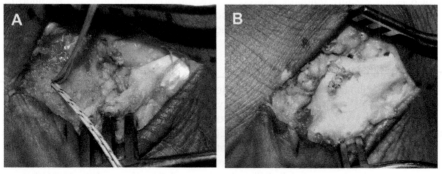

Fig. 3. (*A*) A double-limbed suture anchor placed in the medial cancellous surface of the navicular after excision of the accessory ossicle. (*B*) Posterior tibialis tendon advanced to cancellous surface with sutures limbs.

advancement.[7,19] These tended to be in younger populations of athletes, however, and did not routinely show any improvement in radiographic parameters.[7,19]

Percutaneous drilling of the accessory navicular and synchondrosis in pediatric athletes has been described.[11] This demonstrated return to sports on average at 2 months. Excellent outcomes were obtained in 79% of athletes, with 17% demonstrating good and 3% demonstrating fair results.[11] In 58% of cases, radiographs indicated full healing and union of the accessory bone to the navicular. The investigators felt that younger pediatric athletes with open physes (particularly the hallux proximal phalanx) predicted better outcomes with this approach.[11] There was no assessment, however, of any improvement in radiographic alignment of the foot.[11]

Formal open fusion of the accessory bone to the main body of the navicular has also been described.[20] It was theorized that tendon-to-bone healing may not have sufficient strength particularly in adults, so fusion of the accessory ossicle to the main navicular might produce improved results.[20] This required removal of the synchondrosis tissue as well as flattening down of the medial edge of the native navicular. The accessory bone was then advanced plantar and distal and secured with 1 or 2 small-diameter screws.[10,20] These individuals were immobilized in a cast for 6 weeks followed by a boot for 6 weeks. Case reports have shown union rates at only 82%, however, and almost a quarter of patients had poor results and some limitation with sports.[10] It remains unclear if this offers advantages compared with the modified Kidner procedure, especially in athletes.

Associated procedures such as a gastrocnemius recession or Achilles tendon lengthening are appropriate when the athlete has gastrocnemius or Achilles contracture. Numerous series have shown that addressing the accessory navicular and posterior tibial tendon attachment site alone without any associated bony work does not produce improvement in arch alignment.[2,6,9,15] Several level IV series have described various realignment procedures in conjunction with a modified Kidner procedure. One technique recommended a subtalar arthroereisis implant to improve hindfoot and arch alignment in conjunction with a modified Kidner procedure[9] (**Fig. 4**). A portion of these individuals also had a gastrocnemius recession. This study noted improved VAS pain and clinical outcome scores as well as improved alignment including Meary angle and talonavicular coverage.[9] This had high satisfaction rates, although 15% did require later removal of the arthroereisis implant.[9] Other investigators have reported use of medial displacement calcaneal osteotomy to improve hindfoot alignment in conjunction with the modified Kidner procedure[18] (**Fig. 5**). This comprised an older population including adults as old as 64. This approach yielded improved American Orthopaedic Foot & Ankle Society outcome scores and radiographic parameters.[18] Addition of cuboid and cuneiform osteotomies in addition to medial displacement calcaneal osteotomy in adolescents showed improved clinical scores and radiographic parameters as well.[21]

Authors' preferred technique

Surgeons have limited clinical data available with which to make evidence-based decisions on the treatment of painful accessory navicular in athletes. Literature on accessory navicular surgery is very heterogeneous, with studies that include both athletes and nonathletes alike as well as patient groups with wide ranging ages. The authors' preferred approach to managing symptomatic athletes is to perform the modified Kidner procedure. In our opinion, this has robust clinical data with good symptomatic relief and reliable healing especially in the athletic population. Our preferred technique is to expose the medial navicular and the posterior tibialis tendon insertion. The interface between the accessory navicular and main navicular can be identified with a scalpel

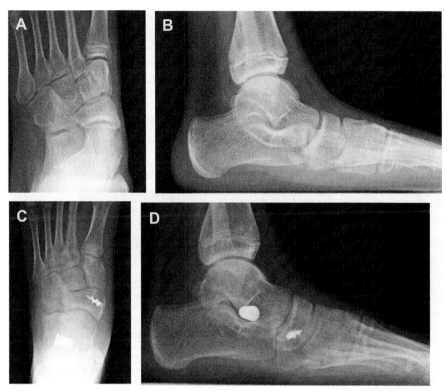

Fig. 4. (*A*) Anteroposterior (AP) and (*B*) lateral radiographs of an adolescent tennis player with painful accessory navicular. (*C*) Postoperative AP and (*D*) lateral radiographs following subtalar arthroereisis implant along with modified Kidner procedure.

blade or hypodermic needle. In some cases the plantar-laterally directed plane of this interface may be difficult to find and the use of intraoperative fluoroscopy can be useful to confirm the position. This plane is then developed and the accessory ossicle carefully shelled out with a scalpel. Care is taken to minimize soft tissue detachment plantarly as the distal fibers of the tendon extend to the cuneiforms. It is essential to remove the excess bone on the medial navicular and the authors prefer a microsagittal saw to provide a smooth cancellous surface for tendon reattachment. Metallic or all-suture anchors can then be inserted under fluoroscopic guidance into the medial navicular. The posterior tibialis tendon insertion is then advanced and tied down to the medial cancellous bone surface, with the ankle held in 10° of plantarflexion and 10° of inversion for proper tensioning. Holding the ankle in maximal inversion during advancement should be avoided to prevent overtightening the tendon.

If the patient has contracture of the gastrocnemius or Achilles, an adjunctive gastrocnemius recession or Achilles tendon lengthening is performed. Patients with concomitant pes planus need correction of the malalignment with bony procedures, as the Kidner procedure alone does not correct alignment. Increased heel valgus is typically addressed with a medial displacement calcaneal osteotomy. The medial displacement calcaneal osteotomy has predictable bone healing and good clinical results with very little impact on subtalar motion. In the setting of severe midfoot abduction and uncoverage of the talonavicular joint, we instead perform a lateral column

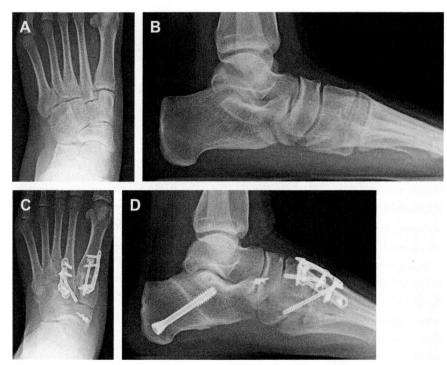

Fig. 5. A college volleyball player with painful Type II accessory navicular following un-treated Lisfranc injury of the midfoot with abduction deformity. (*A*) Preoperative AP and (*B*) lateral radiographs. (*C*) Postoperative AP and (*D*) lateral radiographs following modified Kidner procedure and medializing calcaneal osteotomy combined with corrective arthrod-esis of the Lisfranc injury.

lengthening calcaneal osteotomy with an allograft wedge and screw fixation. This has excellent correction of the hindfoot deformity and reliable healing especially in younger patients. In limited cases, some stiffness of the subtalar joint can occur so it is impor-tant in the athlete not to overlengthen the lateral column or allow graft impingement in the sinus tarsi. A plantarflexion opening wedge osteotomy of the medial cuneiform can also improve arch height. In a very young athlete with open physes and future growth potential, a subtalar arthroereisis can yield good correction of the hindfoot without the need for osteotomies.

Postoperatively the patient is immobilized in a short leg cast or boot for up to 6 weeks to allow osteotomy healing and healing of the posterior tibial tendon to the navicular. Weightbearing is subsequently advanced along with active motion exer-cises and open chain strengthening. Heavier resistance strength training and closed chain exercises commence around 8 to 10 weeks postoperatively. The patient re-sumes sneakers or footwear at approximately 8 to 10 weeks and an orthotic medial arch support can be beneficial. Most young athletes can be expected to return to un-restricted participation by 5 to 6 months after surgery.

SPRING LIGAMENT INJURIES
Introduction

The spring ligament is an important component of the static restraints of the medial longitudinal arch of the foot. This name is actually a misnomer, as histologic studies have shown that the tissue is not springy or elastic but has properties consistent with a typical ligament.[22,23] It is composed of 3 main portions. The superior medial calcaneonavicular (SMCN) bundle is a broad, triangular-shaped ligament that fans out from the anteromedial margin of the sustentaculum of the calcaneus to insert on the navicular margin[22–24] (**Fig. 6**). The SMCN portion also contains an overlying layer of fibrocartilage for articulation with the talar head. The inferior calcaneonavicular (ICN) is a narrow band like, quadrilateral ligament with its origin between the anterior and middle facets of the sustentaculum; it inserts plantarly on the lateral portion of the navicular[22–24] (**Fig. 7**). The medial plantar oblique (MPO) or "third ligament" also originates from the facet between anterior and middle facets of the calcaneus but courses more medially than the ICN, deep to the fibrocartilage of the SMCN[23,24] (**Fig. 8**). Anatomic studies have shown that there is continuity with fibers of the deltoid, specifically the tibiocalcaneonavicular ligament.[25] The spring ligament recess is an outpouching of the plantar capsule of the talonavicular joint between the ICN and MPO portions; this can be misinterpreted on MRI studies as a disruption of the ligaments.[26]

The spring ligament complex acts as a static restraint to the arch, along with the plantar fascia, tibionavicular ligament, long and short plantar ligaments, and the talocalcaneal ligament.[27] The spring ligament acts as a sling for the talar head, the so-called acetabulum pedis, preventing the talar head from plantarflexing.[22,26] Incompetence or injury of the spring ligament may allow subluxation of the talonavicular joint,

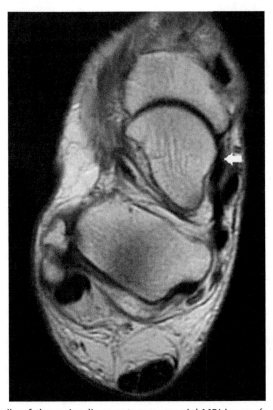

Fig. 6. SMCN bundle of the spring ligament seen on axial MRI image *(arrow)*.

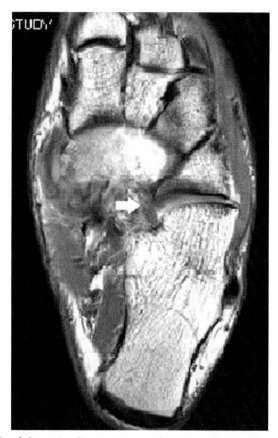

Fig. 7. ICN bundle of the spring ligament on axial MRI image *(arrow).*

wherein the talar head sags into plantarflexion with associated abduction through the transverse tarsal joint and eversion of the calcaneus leading to hindfoot valgus.[26,28]

Clinical Evaluation

Acute isolated injuries of the spring ligament are relatively uncommon. The vast majority of the literature regarding spring ligament injuries focuses on their occurrence in conjunction with chronic degeneration or tearing of the posterior tibialis tendon. That represents a distinct pathologic entity from acute spring ligament injuries in the athletic population. Acute spring ligament injury often results from an abduction or eversion type mechanism during sports.[29,30] An awkward landing from a fall can also injure the spring ligament,[31] and has been described in a pole vaulter landing from a jump.[32] Many athletes have an unclear mechanism of injury and describe a sprain injury. Sports represented in the literature include soccer, track and field, cricket, and tennis, although virtually any running or jumping athlete can sustain this type of injury.[29,30,33]

The clinician should perform a detailed history to identify the mechanism of injury. The athlete's ability to bear weight immediately afterward may correlate with the severity of the ligament disruption. It is important to identify if the athlete notices asymmetric deformity of the foot. Initial treatment by the training staff should be reviewed as

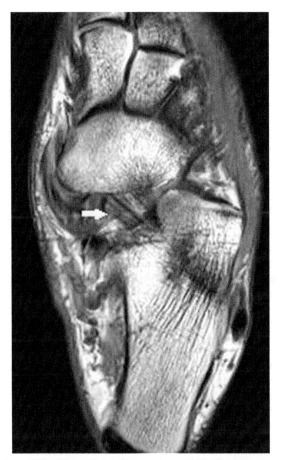

Fig. 8. MPO bundle of the spring ligament on axial MRI image *(arrow)*.

well. On physical examination, the patient will typically present with medial arch swelling.[31,33] Medial tenderness is almost always present,[33] although some patients also have lateral pain and impingement in the sinus tarsi or subfibular region depending on the presence of deformity.[34] Severe rupture of the spring ligament can lead to collapse of the medial longitudinal arch along with abduction ("too many toes") and hindfoot valgus.[29–31] It is critical to evaluate the strength of the posterior tibialis tendon to identify associated tendon injury. Many patients with spring ligament pathology have maintained posterior tibialis tendon strength on manual muscle testing.[29] Single limb heel rise, however, can be difficult and the hindfoot may remain in valgus without appropriate inversion.[29,30,34] It is also necessary to evaluate the degree of flexibility of the hindfoot and identify the presence of Achilles tendon or gastrocnemius contracture.

Standard weightbearing radiographs of the foot are obtained including anteroposterior, lateral, and oblique views. It is also necessary to obtain weightbearing radiographs of the ankle to rule out evidence of deltoid ligament injury, such as medial clear space widening or valgus tilt. The foot radiographs are inspected for evidence of deformity including abduction and uncoverage of the talonavicular joint, loss of the medial longitudinal arch, and dorsal subluxation of the navicular.[29,31,32] The absence of foot deformity clinically and radiographically, of course does not rule out spring ligament injury.

Additional imaging is often necessary to evaluate this injury. MRI is a mainstay in the diagnosis of spring ligament pathology. Previous literature has indicated MRI has a moderate sensitivity of 55% with a high specificity of 100%.[35] Individuals with spring ligament pathology will often show edema in the navicular and possibly the talar head.[32] MRI is very effective at imaging the distal aspect of the posterior tibialis tendon, although many individuals with an isolated spring ligament injury may not have obvious tendon pathology as is typical in more chronic cases of posterior tibialis tendinosis and tearing with secondary ligament failure. The SMCN bundle can be very reliably imaged on MRI scan.[36] It is best seen on axial and coronal cuts and is typically 2 to 3 mm in thickness. The sagittal plane images are somewhat limited in evaluating the SMCN, due to the plantar recess between the bundles that can mimic discontinuity of the ligament. A 50° oblique sagittal view has been described for better visualization.[32] Acute spring ligament tear typically shows high signal intensity on T2 imaging and splitting or discontinuity of the ligament fibers[35] (**Fig. 9**). Chronic injury cases may show heterogeneous or increased signal intensity on T2 images with a thickened (>4 mm) or thinned attenuated (<2 mm) appearance on axial views along with a wavy characteristic.[28,30,35] The ICN bundle is best seen on axial and coronal images and normally shows intermediate signal intensity on T1 and low intensity on T2 images. The MPO or third ligament has a striated appearance on the axial and coronal images. This ligament can be harder to visualize and may be less reliable in the clinical diagnosis.[36]

Ultrasound has also been described as being effective at visualizing the superior medial bundle.[30] Ultrasound can indicate disruption or thickening of the ligament fibers and also allows visualization of the distal aspect of the posterior tibialis tendon. In athletes with isolated spring ligament injury, the posterior tibialis tendon is usually intact with a normal appearance and no obvious thickening or degeneration.[29,30]

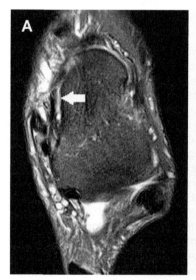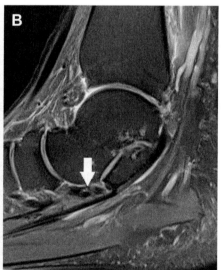

Fig. 9. (*A*) Axial and (*B*) sagittal MRI images showing tearing of SMCN portion of spring ligament (*arrow*).

Nonsurgical Treatment

Nonoperative treatment is appropriate initially in most spring ligament injuries. Protected weightbearing and immobilization is the mainstay of early treatment, along with rest, icing, and nonsteroidal anti-inflammatory drugs for pain relief. As advanced imaging is often necessary, the athlete should be maintained nonweightbearing in a cast or boot until definitive diagnosis can be obtained.[31] Partial injury without arch collapse or foot deformity can be treated nonsurgically, with nonweightbearing for approximately 4 to 6 weeks and then weightbearing progression along with physiotherapy. The patient typically progresses out of the boot over the course of 3 to 4 weeks and a custom molded orthotic arch support is routinely prescribed. In one series, two-thirds of athletes and military recruits were successfully treated with orthotic management.[30] For individuals with complete tear of the ligament complex or resultant foot deformity, surgery is virtually always necessary. Some investigators also recommend surgery in younger patients or athletic individuals as a matter of routine,[30] although literature directly comparing nonoperative and surgical management is extremely limited.

Surgical Decision Making

Solid evidence-based recommendations regarding surgical treatment of spring ligament injuries in athletes is lacking. Most literature regarding spring ligament problems is heavily concerned with older patients with posterior tibialis tendon insufficiency, which comprises a far different patient cohort than athletes. Similarly, literature on isolated spring ligament pathology without associated posterior tibial tendon injuries is sparse. Virtually all reports are Level IV or V retrospective case series.

Most reports discuss primary repair of the spring ligament medially.[32,34,37,38] This included use of nonabsorbable sutures, often in an imbrication or vest-over-pants configuration.[29,30] In some instances, investigators have described advancing ligament fibers to the navicular and attaching them through drill holes in bone.[33]

More recently, augmentation of spring ligament repair with suture tape constructs has been described.[39] This typically involves a bony tunnel in the sustentaculum with a vertical tunnel in the navicular. A suture tape device can be inserted into the sustentaculum tunnel with dorsal and plantar suture tape limbs passed through the navicular tunnel to re-create the configuration of the SMCN ligament. The underlying spring ligament fibers are also repaired. An alternate construct has been described that involves suture tape woven in a figure-of-8 configuration through the navicular and sustentaculum, although robust clinical data and biomechanical analysis are lacking.[40]

Numerous studies have described reconstruction of the spring ligament, as many investigators feel the native tissue may be inadequate for healing following direct repair. It is again critical to recognize that many of these reports deal with an older patient cohort who also have combined degeneration and tearing of the posterior tibialis tendon, so direct comparison to the younger, healthier athletic population may be suspect. Distal advancement of the posterior tibialis tendon has been described in pediatric athletes.[31] Several versions of spring ligament repair with augmentation by posterior tibialis tendon autograft have also been devised.[34,41] This can involve simple suturing of the adjacent stump of the posterior tibial tendon into the spring ligament[34] or more complex fashioning of the distal tendon stump to allow insertion into a drill tunnel in the sustentaculum and fixation with an interference screw.[41] This has shown good correction of deformity including restoration of the Meary angle and talonavicular coverage. It is crucial to recognize that these augmentation procedures require resection of the posterior tibialis tendon and rely on use of diseased tissue, which again may not be relevant in the athletic population in whom the tendon is usually not involved. Other autologous grafts have been described, including use of peroneus longus and flexor hallucis longus tendons.[42,43] Both techniques require sacrifice of their respective donor tendons and then complex 3-dimensional weaving through multiple bone tunnels in the midfoot and sustentaculum to reestablish support of the talar head similar to the native spring ligament. These require sacrificing a normal functioning tendon, which is less than ideal in the high demand sports population. Similarly, flexor digitorum longus transfer has routinely been performed in posterior tibialis tendon insufficiency and may provide some support to the medial arch[29,30]; again, this technique may not be relevant in athletes unless they have an associated posterior tibial tendon tear. Use of allograft tissue may offer an alternative reconstruction option without sacrifice of an autologous donor tendon, but its use in athletes with an intact posterior tibial tendon is rare.

Authors' preferred technique

The authors' approach spring ligament injuries in athletes in an aggressive manner. Careful clinical examination and review of radiographic studies are performed to identify the presence of foot deformity, insufficiency or weakness of the posterior tibialis tendon, and the severity of the injury. Mild sprains are routinely treated nonsurgically with rest, immobilization, and graduated physical therapy, as described previously. In our experience, this represents a minority of patients, as many athletes present with early deformity, severe symptoms, and imaging studies suggestive of complete tear of the ligament. In most cases, we tend to manage the athletic population surgically for more reliable correction, accelerated rehabilitation and return to play, and lower risk of later deformity.

Athletes can be successfully managed in most cases with repair and imbrication of the spring ligament fibers using nonabsorbable suture. If the ligament is avulsed off the navicular insertion, suture anchors can allow reattachment to the bone successfully. In chronic cases or larger athletes, we routinely augment the spring ligament repair with fiber tape as described by Acevedo and Vora.[39] This is a reliable technique that holds up well in athletes and avoids sacrificing normal healthy tendons for autologous graft. We prefer the triangular configuration for this augmentation construct, with an interference screw anchored into the sustentaculum and the dorsal and plantar suture tape limbs passed through a vertical navicular tunnel and secured with a second interference screw (**Fig. 10**). It is essential not to overtighten this, so the repair is secured with the talonavicular joint inverted approximately 5°.

Similar to patients with accessory navicular problems, associated foot deformities should be corrected at the time of soft tissue repair. Contractures of the Achilles tendon or gastrocnemius are corrected with Achilles lengthening or gastrocnemius recession. Any degree of abnormal hindfoot valgus should be addressed with a medial displacement calcaneal osteotomy,[30,37] which has the advantage of providing some protection to soft tissue repairs of the medial column of the arch. In our experience, severe deformities in athletes are relatively uncommon so more advanced flatfoot correction procedures such as lateral column lengthening osteotomy[31,37] or plantarflexion osteotomy of the cuneiform are not necessary.

Patients are routinely kept nonweightbearing for 6 weeks following the medial soft tissue repair and any associated bony procedures. Progressive weightbearing in a fracture boot with a medial wedge then commences and gradually advances to full weightbearing over 3 to 4 weeks. Athletes can work on open chain leg strengthening along with upper extremity and core strengthening and low impact conditioning exercises. In later stages, closed chain exercise progresses followed by advancement to

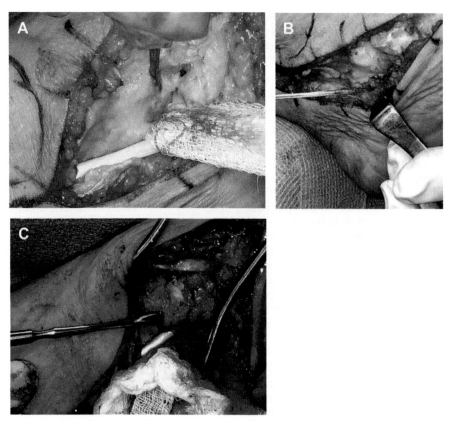

Fig. 10. Preferred technique for spring ligament repair. (*A*) Elevator demonstrating tear in SMCN portion of spring ligament. (*B*) Suture tape inserted into sustentaculum. (*C*) Suture tape limbs inserted through vertical tunnel in navicular, along with flexor digitorum longus transfer in patient with concomitant posterior tibialis tear (elevator indicating dorsal limb of suture tape).

running and cutting beginning 3 months postoperatively. Many patients benefit from a custom molded medial orthotic arch support once they graduate out of a fracture boot; this can be continued once they resume use of their training shoe and sport shoe or cleat.

Rehabilitation Considerations

The athlete presents particular challenges following surgical management. Careful monitoring of the individual's progress during rehabilitation is essential to allow appropriate healing and recovery while expediting return to play. Heavier training and simulated sports activities typically commence between 3 and 4 months postoperatively. Pain-free ambulation along with restored strength and stability are necessary before allowing the athlete to initiate a running protocol. Interval jogging is followed by progressively longer running, sprinting, and explosive movements. Agility training including ladder drills and figure-of-8 running represents a later stage of rehabilitation along with plyometrics and cutting maneuvers. As the athlete makes progress, simulated drills for their particular sport can be incorporated such as throwing, catching, and sport-specific movements. Full return to performance including practice and game play require ongoing monitoring among the surgeon, athletic training staff, and coaching staff to ensure a successful recovery and return to sports.

DISCLOSURE

The authors have nothing to disclose.

REFERENCES

1. Lawson JP, Ogden JA, Sella E, et al. The painful accessory navicular. Skeletal Radiol 1984;12(4):250–62.
2. Veitch JM. Evaluation of the Kidner procedure in treatment of symptomatic accessory tarsal scaphoid. Clin Orthop Relat Res 1978;131:210–3.
3. Kidner FC. The prehallux (accessory scaphoid) in its relation to flat-foot. J Bone Joint Surg 1929;11:831–7.
4. Kidner FC. The prehallux in relation to flatfoot. JAMA 1933;11:1539–42.
5. Sullivan JA, Miller WA. The relationship of the accessory navicular to the development of the flat foot. Clin Orthop Relat Res 1979;(144):233–7.
6. Prichasuk S, Sinphurmsukskul O. Kidner procedure for symptomatic accessory navicular and its relation to pes planus. Foot Ankle Int 1995;16(8):500–3.
7. Pretell-Mazzini JM RF, Sawyer JR, Spence DD, et al. Surgical treatment of symptomatic accessory navicular in children and adolescents. Am J Orthop 2014; 43(3):110–3.
8. Jegal H, Park YU, Kim JS, et al. Accessory navicular syndrome in athlete vs general population. Foot Ankle Int 2016;37(8):862–7.
9. Garras DN, Hansen PL, Miller AG, et al. Outcome of modified Kidner procedure with subtalar arthroereisis for painful accessory navicular associated with planovalgus deformity. Foot Ankle Int 2012;33(11):934–9.
10. Chung JW, Chu IT. Outcome of fusion of a painful accessory navicular to the primary navicular. Foot Ankle Int 2009;30(2):106–9.
11. Nakayama S, Sugimoto K, Takakura Y, et al. Percutaneous drilling of symptomatic accessory navicular in young athletes. Am J Sports Med 2005;33(4):531–5.
12. Seehausen DA, Harris LR, Kay RM, et al. Accessory navicular is associated with wider and more prominent navicular bone in pediatric patients by radiographic measurement. J Pediatr Orthop 2016;36(5):521–5.
13. Sella EJ, Lawson JP, Ogden JA. The accessory navicular synchondrosis. Clin Orthop Relat Res 1986;209:280–5.
14. Miller TT, Staron RB, Feldman F, et al. The symptomatic accessory tarsal navicular bone: assessment with MR imaging. Radiology 1995;195(3):849–53.
15. Kopp FJ, Marcus RE. Clinical outcome of surgical treatment of the symptomatic accessory navicular. Foot Ankle Int 2004;25(1):27–30.
16. Lee KT, Kim KC, Park YU, et al. Midterm outcome of modified Kidner procedure. Foot Ankle Int 2012;33(2):122–7.
17. Scott AT, Sabesan VJ, Saluta JR, et al. Fusion versus excision of the symptomatic Type II accessory navicular: a prospective study. Foot Ankle Int 2009;30(1):10–5.
18. Cao HH, Tang KL, Lu WZ, et al. Medial displacement calcaneal osteotomy with posterior tibial tendon reconstruction for the flexible flatfoot with symptomatic accessory navicular. J Foot Ankle Surg 2014;53(5):539–43.
19. Cha SM, Shin HD, Kim KC, et al. Simple excision vs the Kidner procedure for type 2 accessory navicular associated with flatfoot in pediatric population. Foot Ankle Int 2013;34(2):167–72.

20. Malicky ES, Levine DS, Sangeorzan BJ. Modification of the Kidner procedure with fusion of the primary and accessory navicular bones. Foot Ankle Int 1999; 20(1):53–4.
21. Kim JR, Park CI, Moon YJ, et al. Concomitant calcaneo-cuboid-cuneiform osteotomies and the modified Kidner procedure for severe flatfoot associated with symptomatic accessory navicular in children and adolescents. J Orthop Surg Res 2014;9:131.
22. Davis WH, Sobel M, DiCarlo EF, et al. Gross, histological, and microvascular anatomy and biomechanical testing of the spring ligament complex. Foot Ankle Int 1996;17(2):95–102.
23. Taniguchi A, Tanaka Y, Takakura Y, et al. Anatomy of the spring ligament. J Bone Joint Surg Am 2003;85(11):2174–8.
24. Patil V, Ebraheim NA, Frogameni A, et al. Morphometric dimensions of the calcaneonavicular (spring) ligament. Foot Ankle Int 2007;28(8):927–32.
25. Cromeens BP, Kirchhoff CA, Patterson RM, et al. An attachment-based description of the medial collateral and spring ligament complexes. Foot Ankle Int 2015; 36(6):710–21.
26. Desai KR, Beltran LS, Bencardino JT, et al. The spring ligament recess of the talocalcaneonavicular joint: depiction on MR images with cadaveric and histologic correlation. AJR Am J Roentgenol 2011;196(5):1145–50.
27. Kitaoka HB, Ahn TK, Luo ZP, et al. Stability of the arch of the foot. Foot Ankle Int 1997;18(10):644–8.
28. Toye LR, Helms CA, Hoffman BD, et al. MRI of spring ligament tears. AJR Am J Roentgenol 2005;184(5):1475–80.
29. Borton DC, Saxby TS. Tear of the plantar calcaneonavicular (spring) ligament causing flatfoot. A case report. J Bone Joint Surg Br 1997;79(4):641–3.
30. Tryfonidis M, Jackson W, Mansour R, et al. Acquired adult flat foot due to isolated plantar calcaneonavicular (spring) ligament insufficiency with a normal tibialis posterior tendon. Foot Ankle Surg 2008;14(2):89–95.
31. Shuen V, Prem H. Acquired unilateral pes planus in a child caused by a ruptured plantar calcaneonavicular (spring) ligament. J Pediatr Orthop B 2009;18(3): 129–30.
32. Chen JP, Allen AM. MR diagnosis of traumatic tear of the spring ligament in a pole vaulter. Skeletal Radiol 1997;26(5):310–2.
33. Masaragian HJ, Ricchetti HO, Testa C. Acute isolated rupture of the spring ligament: a case report and review of the literature. Foot Ankle Int 2013;34(1):150–4.
34. Gazdag AR, Cracchiolo A 3rd. Rupture of the posterior tibial tendon. Evaluation of injury of the spring ligament and clinical assessment of tendon transfer and ligament repair. J Bone Joint Surg Am 1997;79(5):675–81.
35. Yao L, Gentili A, Cracchiolo A. MR imaging findings in spring ligament insufficiency. Skeletal Radiol 1999;28(5):245–50.
36. Williams G, Widnall J, Evans P, et al. MRI features most often associated with surgically proven tears of the spring ligament complex. Skeletal Radiol 2013;42(7): 969–73.
37. Orr JD, Nunley JA 2nd. Isolated spring ligament failure as a cause of adult-acquired flatfoot deformity. Foot Ankle Int 2013;34(6):818–23.
38. Johnson JE, Cohen BE, DiGiovanni BF, et al. Subtalar arthrodesis with flexor digitorum longus transfer and spring ligament repair for treatment of posterior tibial tendon insufficiency. Foot Ankle Int 2000;21(9):722–9.
39. Acevedo J, Vora A. Anatomical reconstruction of the spring ligament complex: "internal brace" augmentation. Foot Ankle Spec 2013;6(6):441–5.

40. Palmanovich E, Shabat S, Brin YS, et al. Novel reconstruction technique for an isolated plantar calcaneonavicular (SPRING) ligament tear: A 5 case series report. Foot (Edinb) 2017;30:1–4.
41. Ryssman DB, Jeng CL. Reconstruction of the Spring Ligament With a Posterior Tibial Tendon Autograft: Technique Tip. Foot Ankle Int 2017;38(4):452–6.
42. Williams BR, Ellis SJ, Deyer TW, et al. Reconstruction of the spring ligament using a peroneus longus autograft tendon transfer. Foot Ankle Int 2010;31(7):567–77.
43. Lee WC, Yi Y. Spring ligament reconstruction using the autogenous flexor hallucis longus tendon. Orthopedics 2014;37(7):467–71.

Achilles Tendinosis Injuries—Tendinosis to Rupture (Getting the Athlete Back to Play)

Jeffrey Okewunmi, BS, Javier Guzman, MD, Ettore Vulcano, MD*

KEYWORDS

- Tendinosis • Achilles tendon • Insertional Achilles tendinosis
- Noninsertional Achilles tendinosis • Achilles tendon rupture • Return to play

KEY POINTS

- Recreational athletes are susceptible to experiencing pain in the Achilles tendon, affecting their ability to complete daily activities.
- Achilles tendinosis is a degenerative process of the tendon without histologic or clinical signs of intratendinous inflammation, which can be categorized by location into insertional and noninsertional tendinosis.
- This condition is one that can be treated conservatively with great success or surgically for refractory cases.
- Currently, there is a lack of consensus regarding the best treatment options.
- This review aims to explore both conservative and operative treatment options for Achilles tendinopathy and Achilles tendon rupture.

INTRODUCTION

The Achilles tendon, the largest and strongest tendon in the human body, is formed by the inferior tendons of the gastrocnemius and soleus muscles.[1] These tendons join and insert on the posterior aspect of the calcaneus. Achilles tendinosis is a degenerative process of the tendon without histologic or clinical signs of inflammation within the tendon.[2] Degeneration, rather than inflammation, accounts for most intratendinous pain. Achilles tendinosis is frequently seen in athletic populations and is associated with activities that require running and jumping.[3] These activities require strong repetitive toe push-off forces, generating both tensile and torsional forces.[3] Achilles tendinosis is seen most often among recreational male runners aged between 35

Department of Orthopaedic Surgery, Icahn School of Medicine at Mount Sinai, 1 Gustave L. Levy Place, New York, NY 10029, USA
* Corresponding author.
E-mail address: ettore.vulcano@mountsinai.org

Clin Sports Med 39 (2020) 877–891
https://doi.org/10.1016/j.csm.2020.05.001
0278-5919/20/© 2020 Elsevier Inc. All rights reserved.

and 45 years.[1] Most tendon injuries are the result of gradual degeneration from over-use, aging, or a combination of both, stemming from repetitive movements.[2] These areas of tendinosis may eventually progress to partial or complete ruptures if they experience high loads, especially during push-off and landing activities.[4] The assumption is that most ruptures happen only in the setting of previous tendinosis, whether in athletes or the general population.

Achilles tendinosis can be subcategorized based on anatomic location: insertional and noninsertional. Insertional Achilles tendinosis is isolated pain arising at the tendo-Achilles junction, whereas noninsertional Achilles tendinosis is isolated pain arising in the main body of the Achilles, 2 to 6 cm proximal to the Achilles insertion.[3]

The cause of Achilles tendinosis is unclear, but it is likely a multifactorial process, beginning with a mechanical injury stimulus. Tendinosis may either arise from physiologic overloading of the tendon or through an accumulation of multiple physiologic loads without adequate healing.[3] From a cellular perspective, tendinosis is a failure of the cell matrix to adapt to trauma, causing an imbalance between the degeneration and synthesis of the matrix.[3] Hypotheses for factors that cause Achilles tendinosis may be categorized into intrinsic or extrinsic. Intrinsic factors include age, gender, body mass index, biomechanical abnormalities, foot malalignment, gastrocnemius-soleus dysfunction, ankle instability, insufficient blood supply, insufficient tensile strength, muscle imbalance, and insufficient flexibility. Extrinsic factors include over-use, steroid use, fluoroquinolones, improper training, environmental factors, and footwear.[3] Etiologic factors for the development of Achilles tendinosis include aging with a decreased blood supply and decreased tensile strength, muscle weakness and imbalance, insufficient flexibility, male gender, overweight, malalignments, leg length discrepancy, training errors with overloading, improper footwear, systemic diseases, and drug adverse events.[1] Risk factors for this condition may include diabetes, hypertension, obesity, hormone replacement, use of oral contraceptives, and pes cavus.[2]

Most patients with this condition report a gradual onset without trauma.[2] Tendinosis can present as a painless thickening of the Achilles tendon. On gross examination, Achilles tendinosis appears as a yellowish, thickened tendon from the accumulation of mucinous material within the diseased area and it will be tender on palpation.[5] An MRI is useful in determining the extent of intratendinous degeneration.[5]

PATHOPHYSIOLOGY

The Achilles tendon is surrounded by a single layer of paratenon instead of a true synovial sheath.[5] This paratenon is a highly vascularized single layer of fatty areolar tissue, responsible for most of the blood supply to the Achilles tendon. Most blood supply to the tendon enters anteriorly and creates a hypovascular area 2 to 6 cm proximal to the insertion of the tendon on the calcaneus.[5] Subsequently, any injury to the hypovascular tissue has a prolonged healing process.[6] This longer timeline increases the likelihood that damaging forces occur before the tissue can ever fully recover. In the healing process, when tissue breakdown exceeds the repair process, tendinosis occurs.[6]

In a normal Achilles, 90% to 95% of the cellular makeup is tenocytes and tenoblasts. The other cellular components of tendons include chondrocytes, vascular, synovial, and smooth muscle cells.[3] The Achilles tendon extracellular matrix is primarily composed of type I collagen, elastin fibers, ground substance, and organic components, such as calcium.[3] Healing in the Achilles tendon is likely mediated by tenocytes that detect changes within the extracellular matrix.[3] Studies suggest that the failure to restore this extracellular matrix may result in the release of cytokines that further regulate tenocyte activity and prevent proper healing, therefore creating a degenerative spiral.[3]

Under the degenerative processes, the cellular and extracellular composition of tendons change in addition to changes in histologic appearance.[1] Pathologic Achilles tendons can be recognized by abnormalities in collagen fibers, cystic mucoid, tendolipomatosis, deposits of calcium, and vascular changes.[3] Biopsies of diseased tendons display signs of cellular activation evidenced by increased cell numbers, collagen disarray, and neovascularization.[2] Histologically, collagen abnormalities can appear as abnormal variations in collagen fiber diameter, collagen fibers splitting longitudinally, and collagen fiber disintegration. Cystic mucoid changes appear histologically as large mucoid patches and vacuoles between thin collagen fibers. Tendolipomatosis changes appear as lipid cells interspersed within collagen fibers.[3]

INSERTIONAL ACHILLES TENDINOSIS

As mentioned earlier, there are 2 subdivisions that are distinct within the terminology of Achilles tendinosis. Insertional Achilles tendinosis, as its name implies, revolves around issues affecting the Achilles tendon at its insertion. This condition may be secondary to a posterosuperior calcaneal spur or Haglund deformity; however, the presence of a spur does not indicate the tendinopathy has resulted from its presence. Pain may also stem anterior or posterolateral to the tendon insertion, which may indicate retrocalcaneal bursitis. Although these are different processes, they can occur in concert with insertional tendinopathy.[7] It is hypothesized that because there is dorsiflexion of the ankle, the Achilles tendon experiences attritional microtears as it comes in contact with a Haglund deformity. Moreover, retrocalcaneal bursal hypertrophy and inflammation may further exacerbate the cellular degenerative cascade.[8]

Examination

- Decreased passive dorsiflexion
- Pain with passive and active dorsiflexion/plantarflexion at the extreme range of motion
- Tenderness to palpation at the insertion of the Achilles tendon
- Palpable prominence at the posterosuperior calcaneus
- Hypertrophy or thickening of the tendon at its insertion
- Difficulty with push-off exercises

Imaging

Although the diagnosis of insertional tendinopathy is clinical, radiographs may help to confirm the diagnosis. Weight-bearing (WB) lateral ankle films are the study of choice, as they can identify small bone spurs within the tendon, which suggests a degenerative process. A Haglund deformity may or may not be present. The measuring of Bohler angle, parallel pitch sign, or Fowler-Phillip angle have not been found to correlate with symptomatic Haglund.[9]

NONINSERTIONAL ACHILLES TENDINOSIS

Noninsertional Achilles tendinosis occurs 2 to 6 cm proximal to its insertion and is distinct from insertional Achilles tendinosis. There is typically no calcaneal spur, and the pathology is primarily intratendinous (**Fig. 1**).

Examination

- Pain localized 2 to 6 cm proximal to the calcaneal insertion. Discomfort in this region is increased at the start and end of exercise, with an intermediate period of minimized discomfort.

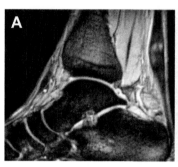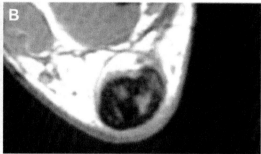

Fig. 1. (*A*) Noninsertional Achilles tendinosis. T2 sagittal MRI of ankle demonstrating thickening and bulbous appearance of Achilles tendon proximal to insertion site. (*B*) Noninsertional Achilles tendinosis. T2 axial MRI through Achilles tendon at painful segment showing heterogeneous appearance of tendon signifying a degenerative and disorganized process.

- Tendon asymmetry, thickening, and scarring.
- Fusiform swelling of the Achilles tendon can be found 2 to 6 cm proximal to the calcaneal insertion.
- Tendon tenderness to palpation, heat, thickening, nodularity, or crepitus.
- Painful plantar flexion and dorsiflexion and nodule movement within the paratenon.

Imaging

Appropriate imaging is helpful in diagnosing and determining a treatment plan. Plain WB lateral radiograph is able to show any intrasubstance calcification, which is helpful in localizing noninsertional Achilles tendinosis. MRI or ultrasound can be used to gather morphologic details on internal tendon morphology and are usually ordered for research purposes, as the diagnosis is typically clinical. On imaging, tendinosis appears as intrasubstance intermediate signal intensity because of the disorganized tissue.

NONOPERATIVE TREATMENT OF ACHILLES TENDINOPATHIES

Noninvasive, conservative methods remain the initial response to the treatment of this condition. For Achilles tendinopathies, treatments such as activity modification, orthotics, heel lifts, massage, hot and cold compresses, strengthening exercises, ultrasound, nonsteroidal antiinflammatory drugs (NSAIDs), and oral corticosteroid are methods that have historically been used.[2] Because of the lack of inflammatory mediators in Achilles tendinosis, the use of NSAIDs and corticosteroids as treatment options has been questioned. Although many of these noninvasive treatments provide patients with short-term pain relief, 25% to 30% of patients find this method of treatment inadequate.[1,2]

Eccentric training, developed by Alfredson and colleagues, is a treatment that promotes tendon healing by increasing tendon volume.[10] After 12 weeks of eccentric training, ultrasound and MRI display a decrease in size and a more normal tendon appearance.[11] Continuous eccentric loading lengthens the muscle-tendon unit and increases the ability for the tendon to bear load over time.[2] Studies evaluating Alfredson's 12-week eccentric training treatment found that this method produced 90% good results with noninsertional Achilles tendinosis and 30% good results with insertional Achilles tendinosis.[12]

Sclerosing agents are a treatment option to reduce pain in patients. By blocking the process of neovascularization in the injured tendon, the sensory nerves associated with blood vessels are also eliminated, which produces pain relief.[12] Polidocanol is a treatment option used to sclerose neovascularization in the Achilles tendon, causing thrombosis through a selective effect on the intima. The Polidocanol treatment protocol is an injection of the sclerosing agent 2 to 3 times, followed by rest without high-impact activities, 6 to 8 weeks apart.[13] There have been occurrences where elite athletes who received Polidocanol treatment, however, have ruptured tendons later in their careers. Sclerosing thermal therapy is another sclerosing agent technique that uses a radiofrequency probe to carry out microtenotomies using thermal energy.[14] Prolotherapy is the use of hypertonic glucose with lignocaine or lidocaine injection designed to sclerose the new blood vessels and nerves. A study showed that the combination of prolotherapy and eccentric loading produced more rapid symptom improvement than eccentric loading alone.[15]

Glyceryl trinitrate is a prodrug, commercially available topical patch that relieves pain through the use of nitric oxide. Nitric oxide is a second messenger that can affect tendon healing by increasing collagen production by fibroblasts, cellular adhesion, and local vascularity.[16] Studies have produced conflicting reports about the results of glyceryltrinitrate use in treatment, so further evaluation is required.

When applied to a diseased tendon, low-level laser therapy can enhance adenosine triphosphate production, enhance cell function, increase protein synthesis, reduce inflammation, increase collagen synthesis, and promote angiogenesis.[17] Limited data suggest that combining low-level laser therapy with eccentric exercises produce decreased pain intensity, morning stiffness, tenderness to palpation, active dorsiflexion, and crepitus with minimal to no side effects.[17]

In chronic Achilles tendinosis, there are fewer platelets, whose role is to produce growth factors that aid in the healing process.[18] An increase in platelet quantity enhances healing in the tissue by stimulating revascularization. There is currently no indication for the use of platelet-rich plasma in Achilles tendinosis, but evidence suggests that improvement is not significantly better than physical therapy.[19]

Extracorporeal shock wave therapy (ESWT) is another viable treatment option, although not yet approved for the treatment of insertional and noninsertional Achilles tendinosis by the Food and Drug Administration. ESWT options include low-energy treatment in 3 weekly sessions without local anesthesia or intravenous anesthesia and high-energy treatment in a single session requiring local or intravenous anesthesia. Repeated shock waves to the affected area cause microtrauma, which then stimulates neovascularization. Neovascularization promotes tissue healing and pain relief. It also has the effect of inhibiting afferent pain receptor function and increasing nitric oxide synthase production. Clinical trials of this treatment option have produced conflicting reports regarding the efficacy of this treatment.[12,20,21]

As there is a multitude of nonoperative treatments for chronic Achilles tendinopathies, it may benefit the patient to trial one or several modalities at the discretion of the surgeon. This may also be limited to the surgeon's accessibility to facilities that are capable of performing some of the nonoperative techniques.

OPERATIVE OPTIONS FOR NONINSERTIONAL ACHILLES TENDINOSIS

Operative Achilles tendinosis treatment involves the removal of abnormal tissues and lesions, fenestration of the tendon through multiple longitudinal creations, and possibly stripping the paratenon. The goal of this treatment is to remove degenerative nodules, excise fibrotic adhesions, restore the vascularity, and stimulate viable cells to initiate an inflammatory response and reinitiate healing.[2] The ultimate goal is to restore the function and strength of the Achilles tendon.

Testa developed a surgical technique where multiple percutaneous incisions are made through the affected Achilles tendon.[22] In this technique, the patient is placed in the prone position, and local anesthesia is applied to the affected area, which can be determined through palpation or ultrasound. A longitudinal incision is made parallel to the long axis of the Achilles tendon using a stab knife. With the knife pointing cephalad, the ankle is then fully dorsiflexed. Then with the scalpel pointing toward the caudal direction, the ankle is then fully plantarflexed. Four separate stab incisions are made approximately 2 cm apart: medial proximal and distal as well as lateral proximal and distal. These incisions are then closed with adhesive strips. Postoperatively, early range of motion is encouraged, and full WB is allowed after 2 to 3 days. The patient is expected to return to their previous activity level after 4 to 6 weeks. Using this procedure, Testa and Maffulli achieved excellent results in 56% of cases, compared with poor results in 8% of cases.[22,23] Later, Maffulli modified technique by adding another stab wound at the central portion of the affected area.[24]

Longo introduced a technique of stripping the adhesions in the Achilles tendon through a minimally invasive technique.[25] This surgical technique involves four 0.5 cm longitudinal skin incisions along the border of the Achilles tendon: 2 just medial and lateral to the origin of the tendon and 2 incisions at the distal end of the tendon close to the insertion. A mosquito is then inserted through the incisions to free the proximal and distal portions of the Achilles tendon of any peritendinous adhesions. A number 1 Ethibond suture is inserted at the 2 proximal incisions over the anterior aspect of the Achilles tendon. Ends of the Ethibond are then retrieved from the distal incisions. The Ethibond is then slid onto the tendon, causing it to be stripped and freed from adhesions at the anterior surface of the tendon. The procedure is repeated for the posterior aspect of the tendon. Theoretically, this will disrupt the neovascularization of the damaged tendon and its accompanying nerve supply. After the procedure, the patient is allowed to do range-of-motion exercises and can be allowed to do full WB.[24]

In endoscopic tendon debridement, small skin incisions are made, and an arthroscopic shaver is introduced into the Achilles tendon to debris the peritenon. This procedure has some evidence that it decreases postoperative complications, thus allowing the patient early return to previous activity.[26] In one study, this procedure produced significant pain relief lasting from 2 to 7 years in 20 patients, who returned to sports after 4 to 6 weeks. Another 5-year follow-up study showed no infection and systemic complications in patients with Achilles tendinosis after this procedure.[27]

In cases of moderate to severe tendinosis or when conservative techniques have been unsuccessfully applied, more invasive open tendon debridement and repair with or without augmentation is an operative option. However, contraindications for this technique are minimal preoperative pain or skin and vascular compromise, and there are reports of tendon rupture after an open debridement. In this operation, the paratenon is incised and any inflamed and any peritendinous tissue is removed. If on MRI or ultrasound there is an intratendinous nodule, or there is a palpable thickening within the tendon, excision is recommended until viable tissues are seen, as residual degenerated tissue increases the risk of persistent postoperative pain.[28]

OPERATIVE OPTIONS FOR INSERTIONAL ACHILLES TENDINOSIS

There are a variety of treatment options; however, most techniques involve excision of the calcaneal spur and debridement of diseased tendon.[29–31] In general, a longitudinal medial or lateral midline incision is made. Careful dissection through the paratenon is performed and any adhesions are freed. The tendon is then detached from its insertion. Once the tendon has been detached from its insertion, all diseased tendons are debrided and calcaneal spur can be taken down with the use of a burr or removed with osteotomes. The retrocalcaneal bursa is debrided at this time. The tendon is then reattached to its insertion using bone anchors. The flexor hallucis longus can be used to augment the Achilles tendon by tendon transfer if more than 50% of the diseased tendon was removed. Some have also advocated the use of the plantaris in cases or excessive debridement.

Postoperative patients are placed in a resting equinus splint for 2 weeks non-WB (NWB) until the wound has healed. The patient is then placed in a WB boot with a heel lift for 6 weeks, and ankle range of motion is allowed. After 6 weeks the patient is allowed to start strengthening. The patient will be allowed a gradual return to sports at 3 months time.

Another surgical option is a dorsal closing wedge calcaneal osteotomy or Zadek osteotomy. The procedure shortens the Achilles tendon to induce a mechanical advantage, consequently alleviating pain and permitting a faster recovery.[32] The osteotomy reduces anterior impingement of the tendon on the superior angle of the posterior calcaneal tuberosity. A dorsal wedge is removed in both cases anterior to the calcaneus with care not to disrupt the plantar hinge. The hinge is closed and screws are used to stabilize the osteotomy (**Fig. 2**). Patients are made NWB for 2 weeks until healing of the wound and allowed to weight bear at 2 weeks in a postoperative boot. Strengthening is started at 2 weeks. In a recent study by the senior author on chronic insertional Achilles tendinopathy treated with percutaneous Zadek osteotomy, a significant improvement in preoperative to postoperative Foot Function Index and visual analogue scale was observed. The overall rate of satisfaction after surgery was 92%. The relief from pain was achieved after an average period of 12 weeks.[33]

Acute Achilles Rupture

The cause of Achilles tendon rupture is multifactorial, and among these factors, sports-related factors are predominant.[34] Because the number of people participating in recreational and competitive sports has increased, the incidence of Achilles tendon rupture has also increased.[34] This rupture most commonly occurs in a noninsertional

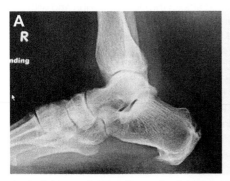
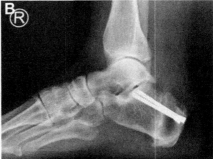

Fig. 2. (A) Lateral WB radiograph of right ankle in patient with insertional Achilles tendinosis. (B) Lateral WB radiograph of right ankle in patient post-Zadek osteotomy. Dorsal wedge osteotomy was closed with 2 partially threaded cancellous screws starting at the posterior aspect of the calcaneus and directed to toward the subtalar joint without intraarticular violation.

area, 2 to 6 cm proximal to the calcaneal insertion.[35] The mechanism of injury is classified into 3 categories: WB with the forefoot pushing off and the knee extended, unanticipated dorsiflexion of the ankle, and violent dorsiflexion of a plantarflexed foot.[36] Although Achilles tendon rupture is considered an acute process, histologic analysis has demonstrated that degenerative changes typical of Achilles tendinosis are commonly found within ruptured tendons.[34] Therefore, Achilles tendinosis is thought to be a factor associated with Achilles tendon rupture.

Examination

Patient history of an acute Achilles tendon rupture is generally straightforward, typically involving a report of a pop, snap, or crack and a sensation of being hit in the area of the rupture.[37] Patients report weakness, poor balance, and altered gait.[38]

The physical examination of Achilles tendon rupture may pose diagnostic challenges. On examination of the tendon, it is not atypical for patients to not report pain.[39] Furthermore, the patient may not exhibit an altered gait because of the recruitment of other extrinsic and intrinsic muscles to assist with plantar flexion. Surrounding swelling and herniation of fat into the rupture space may make palpation difficult, and in neglected ruptures older than 4 weeks, hematoma replacement with healing tendon tissue can "obliterate" the gap.[40]

Several diagnostic tests have been described to diagnose Achilles tendon rupture, which may help minimize missed diagnoses. The calf-squeeze test, described by Simmonds and Thompson, is performed with the patient prone on the examination table with ankles clear of the end of the table or with the knees flexed and feet hanging free at the end of a chair.[41,42] In this position, the examiner squeezes the calf, causing the deformation of the soleus muscle with concurrent posterior bowstringing of the tendon away from the tibia.[43] If there is plantarflexion of the foot, the test is negative (Negative Thompson Test). If the foot remains in neutral or there is minimal plantarflexion compared with the unaffected foot, the test is positive indicating the presence of an Achilles tendon rupture (positive Thompson test). With this technique, Maffulli reported a sensitivity of 0.96 and specificity of 0.93.[40] A false-negative for this test is more likely with a neglected rupture in which hematoma has been replaced with healing tendon tissues.

The knee flexion test, or passive ankle dorsiflexion test, as described by Matles, is performed with the patient prone.[44] In this position, the patient actively flexes the knee to 90°, and the examiner observes both feet and ankles throughout flexion and with the tibia vertical. With an intact tendon, the examiner should observe slight plantarflexion. In contrast, if there is a rupture the affected foot will fall into neutral or slight dorsiflexion. Maffulli reported a sensitivity of 0.88 and a specificity of 0.85 with this test. A neglected rupture still yields a positive result with the knee flexion test, as the tendon will lengthen with hematoma formation and subsequent tendon reconstitution.[40]

The diagnosis of subcutaneous Achilles tendon rupture can reliably be diagnosed with a combination of the calf-squeeze and knee flexion test.[40,45] The American Academy of Orthopedic Surgeons (AAOS) requires findings consistent with rupture in 2 or more of the following tests for clinical diagnosis of Achilles tendon rupture: calf-squeeze test, palpable gap, knee flexion test, or decreased plantarflexion strength.

IMAGING

The diagnosis of the rupture should be clinical. Radiographs can be performed with the lateral ankle projections used to assess Achilles tendon rupture. Loss of normal fat contours or soft tissue density within the normal radiopaque Kager triangle may suggest Achilles tendon rupture. In addition, a positive Arner sign and a decreased Toygar angle indicate an Achilles tendon rupture. A positive Arner sign is when the Achilles tendon deviates anteriorly and no longer parallels the skin surface.[36] The Toygar angle is the ankle of the posterior skin adjacent to the Achilles tendon, and the angle of the skin at the posterior leg overlying the Achilles tendon should be greater than 150°.[46] Another important use of a standard radiograph is to evaluate for any avulsed bone from the calcaneus in the setting of an avulsion-type rupture of the Achilles tendon.

Ultrasound has also been described for use in the assessment of Achilles tendon rupture. The recommended technique is performed with the patient in a prone position with the foot hanging off the edge of the table. The transducer should be set to at least 10 MHz. The transducer is placed in the sagittal plane with observation from the insertion into the calcaneus proximal to the myotendinous junction, then turned 90° for evaluation in the transverse plane. The Achilles tendon should be uniform in thickness and show echogenicity in the longitudinal plane. There should be a hypoechoic ribbonlike image between 2 hyperechoic bands, which should be predominately flat or have a concave anterior margin in the transverse plane. Dynamic imaging can be conducted by gently plantarflexing the foot or with the calf-squeeze test.[47] In areas of rupture, one can observe an "acoustic vacuum" with thick irregular edges at the area of rupture.[48]

MRI is a useful imaging modality to study soft tissue injuries. Typically, the Achilles tendon produces a hypointense signal with all imaging sequences. However, tears show a high T2-weighted signal within the tendon and a focal area of signal intensity at the site of rupture where edema and hemorrhage have collected. Retraction of free ends can occur in acute Achilles tendon tears with T1-weighted signal disruption throughout the tendon itself.[38] MRI study showed a sensitivity of 90%.[49]

The AAOS describes the use of imaging modalities, including radiograph, ultrasound, and MRI, to diagnose Achilles tendon rupture as inconclusive.[50] In patients with the calf-squeeze test, knee flexion test, and palpable gap test indicating Achilles tendon rupture, the findings were confirmed intraoperatively with a sensitivity of 100%. With such sensitive clinical examinations, it is recommended additional imaging be performed only when diagnosis with clinical findings is equivocal. In general, acute Achilles tendon ruptures do not need imaging for diagnosis. In chronic cases, imaging may be useful for clinical planning as retraction may dictate surgical options.

TREATMENT OPTIONS

Although the ruptured tendon can be treated with surgical and nonsurgical therapies, no consensus has yet been reached regarding the optimal treatment protocol. Management of Achilles tendon rupture depends on surgeon and patient preference, with the goal of treatment to restore a normal-length tension relationship, optimizing strength and function while balancing these goals with the known complications of treatment.[51] There lacks a consensus on the patient outcomes of conservative versus surgical repair.

Benefits of surgical repair include alignment of the torn tendon, early active mobilization, and excellent functional results with less chance of rerupture and superior strength, whereas the main disadvantage of open repair is the risk of wound complications.[52] Conservative management leads to tendon healing with extensive scarring, which may lead to lengthening of the tendon and subsequently suboptimal push-off strength.[52]

Different open operative techniques can be used to repair ruptured Achilles tendons ranging from end-to-end suturing by Bunnell- or Kessler-type sutures to more complex repairs using fascial reinforcement or tendon grafts, artificial tendon implants, materials such as absorbable polymer-carbon fiber composites, Marlex mesh, and collagen tendon prostheses.[52] Primary augmentation of the repair with the plantaris tendon, the peroneus brevis tendon, or a single central or 2 (1 medial, 1 lateral) gastrocnemius fascial turndown flap has also been proposed. However, there is no evidence that, in acute AT ruptures, this is better than a nonaugmented end-to-end repair[52] (**Fig. 3**).

With the advent of modern minimally invasive fixation, there have been excellent results with decreased incidence of typical complications such as wound dehiscence and sural nerve injury. This may be particularly useful when treating patients that have poor protoplasm (diabetes, chronic kidney disease, immunosuppressed patients). In addition, modern minimally invasive fixation systems can be used for nearly all patients including athletes with excellent results.[53,54] After undergoing minimally invasive fixation, patients should be placed in an early functional rehab protocol with early WB, starting immediately postoperatively, or shortly after the wound has healed. This, in combination with early active range of motion of the ankle, has superior results to other traditional rehabilitation protocols, with patients returning to

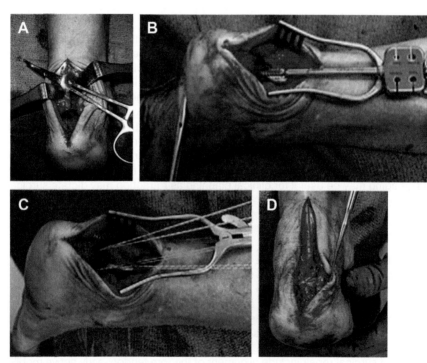

Fig. 3. (*A–D*) Open chronic Achilles tendon rupture repair with flexor hallucis longus (FHL) transfer. (*A*) Achilles tendon has been debrided and FHL tendon has been identified. (*B*) After acquiring maximal length and releasing the FHL tendon, tenodesis screw is used for FHL transfer. (*C*) Suture anchors are placed in preparation for Achilles tendon repair back to its insertion site. (*D*) Achilles tendon has been repaired back to insertion site on calcaneus along with FHL transfer.

preinjury activities, regaining strength, and an excellent range of motion outcomes than patients who undergo prolonged immobilization.[55]

The conclusions of most early studies observing surgical versus conservative treatment were that surgery provides a lower risk of rerupture with higher complication rates. Conservative treatment has gained increasing support with the advent of functional rehabilitation protocol. These protocols demonstrate decreased rerupture rates than cast immobilization but slightly increased rerupture rates when compared with surgery.[56] Functional rehab protocols have decreased complication rates when compared with operative treatment; however, no studies have demonstrated functional rehab to be superior in younger athletic patients. The athlete or active young worker must return to play or work within a reasonable time period with little to no perceptive difference between preinjury and postinjury strength or range of motion.[57] Surgical repair may ensure with more certainty that the tendons are reapproximated appropriately and repaired to allow the tendon to heal with the correct tension, which may subsequently lead to retention of strength. If a conservative approach is to be taken, it is important to note that unless functional rehab is initiated within a reasonable time period after injury (most studies had an inclusion criteria of no more than 5 days postinjury to qualify for nonoperative management), the benefits with regard to rerupture and restoration of function may be lost, and thus if patients present to the surgeon 5 days after injury it may be prudent to discuss surgery.[58] Use of ultrasound or MRI to determine tendon apposition in plantarflexion should be considered before initiation of nonoperative management in all patients, more critically in patients who present after 5 days from injury.

RETURN TO PLAY IN ATHLETES

An Achilles tendon rupture in an athlete can be a potentially devastating injury for a high-level athlete. There is a significant portion of athletes who may not be able to return to play after a repair, as high as 30% in one study, and a clear decline in performance in those that do return to play.[59] The average time to return to play is variable for athletes but can range anywhere from 6 months to 10 months.[60] Whether the patient undergoes open versus minimally invasive repair of the tendon for an acute rupture, it is expected that these athletes will have some worsening of their isometric gastric-soleus strength on the operated side compared with the nonoperated side.[61] A strength decrease of 10% or slightly more may seem inconsequential and possibly imperceivable to some athletes, but it may prove to be a source of decreased performance in particular elite athletes.[62] Moreover, in young athletic patients, there is an increased risk of rerupture, which may be secondary to abnormally large forces placed on the tendon by this patient population.[63] There is no clear consensus or guidelines with regard to optimizing a patient to return to play; however, it is evident that patients who undergo surgery should undergo an early WB and functional rehabilitation protocol to maximize outcomes. Surgeons should limit high-impact activities until the patient is able to progress into normal daily activities without any issues. Once high-impact and push-off activities are initiated, they need to be progressed in a stepwise fashion. Ultimately, there may be a role for a prolonged time to return to play to allow for complete tendon healing and reorganization. Extended time off full play may also allow for any compensatory flexor hallucis longus hypertrophy to occur and further proprioceptive training to be completed by the patient. Earlier return to play must be weighed against the overall potential longevity of the athlete in their respective sport, and it is a decision to be taken on a case-by-case basis. Recently, there has been emerging evidence that nonoperative treatment with functional rehab may also be an option for athletes. Krause and colleagues demonstrated that 67% of high-level athletes were able to return to previous activity at a 5-year follow-up in their cohort of patients. Because new evidence further elucidates nonoperative management protocols, there may also be a role for nonoperative treatment in the cohort of patients who are considered higher-level athletes.[64]

REFERENCES

1. Alfredson H, Lorentzon R. Chronic Achilles tendinosis: recommendations for treatment and prevention. Sports Med 2000;29(2):135–46.
2. Lopez RG, Jung HG. Achilles tendinosis: treatment options. Clin Orthop Surg 2015;7(1):1–7.
3. Singh A, Calafi A, Diefenbach C, et al. Noninsertional Tendinopathy of the Achilles. Foot Ankle Clin 2017;22(4):745–60.
4. Krych A, Warren R, Rodeo S. Chronic Achilles tendon injury: an overview. 2011. Available at: https://www.hss.edu/conditions_chronic-achilles-tendon-problems-overview.asp#tendinosis. Accessed October 9, 2019.
5. Weinfeld SB. Achilles tendon disorders. Med Clin North Am 2014;98(2):331–8.
6. Magnan B, Bondi M, Pierantoni S, et al. The pathogenesis of Achilles tendinopathy: a systematic review. Foot Ankle Surg 2014;20(3):154–9.
7. Irwin TA. Current concepts review: insertional achilles tendinopathy. Foot Ankle Int 2010;31(10):933–9.
8. Roche AJ, Calder JD. Achilles tendinopathy: A review of the current concepts of treatment. Bone Joint J 2013;95-B(10):1299–307.
9. Kang S, Thordarson DB, Charlton TP. Insertional Achilles tendinitis and Haglund's deformity. Foot Ankle Int 2012;33(6):487–91.
10. Alfredson H, Pietilä T, Jonsson P, et al. Heavy-load eccentric calf muscle training for the treatment of chronic Achilles tendinosis. Am J Sports Med 1998;26(3):360–6.
11. Shalabi A, Kristoffersen-Wiberg M, Aspelin P, et al. Immediate Achilles tendon response after strength training evaluated by MRI. Med Sci Sports Exerc 2004;36(11):1841–6.
12. Lake JE, Ishikawa SN. Conservative treatment of Achilles tendinopathy: emerging techniques. Foot Ankle Clin 2009;14(4):663–74.
13. Alfredson H, Ohberg L, Forsgren S. Is vasculo-neural ingrowth the cause of pain in chronic Achilles tendinosis? An investigation using ultrasonography and colour Doppler, immunohistochemistry, and diagnostic injections. Knee Surg Sports Traumatol Arthrosc 2003;11(5):334–8.
14. Boesen M, Torp-Pedersen S, Koenig M, et al. Ultrasound guided electrocoagulation in patients with chronic non-insertional Achilles tendinopathy: a pilot study. Br J Sports Med 2006;40(9):761–6.
15. Yelland M, Sweeting K, Lyftogt J, et al. Prolotherapy injections and eccentric loading exercises for painful Achilles tendinosis: a randomised trial. Br J Sports Med 2011;45(5):421–8.
16. Murrell GA. Using nitric oxide to treat tendinopathy. Br J Sports Med 2007;41(4):227–31.
17. Stergioulas A, Stergioula M, Aarskog R, et al. Effects of low-level laser therapy and eccentric exercises in the treatment of recreational athletes with chronic achilles tendinopathy. Am J Sports Med 2008;36(5):881–7.
18. Magnussen RA, Dunn WR, Thomson AB. Nonoperative treatment of midportion Achilles tendinopathy: a systematic review. Clin J Sport Med 2009;19(1):54–64.

19. de Jonge S, de Vos R, Weir A, et al. One-year follow-up of platelet-rich plasma treatment in chronic Achilles tendinopathy: a double-blind randomized placebo-controlled trial. Am J Sports Med 2011;39(8):1623–9.

20. Furia JP. High-energy extracorporeal shock wave therapy as a treatment for insertional Achilles tendinopathy. Am J Sports Med 2006;34(5):733–40.

21. Furia JP. High-energy extracorporeal shock wave therapy as a treatment for chronic noninsertional Achilles tendinopathy. Am J Sports Med 2008;36(3):502–8.

22. Testa V, Capasso G, Benazzo F, et al. Management of Achilles tendinopathy by ultrasound-guided percutaneous tenotomy. Med Sci Sports Exerc 2002;34(4):573–80.

23. Maffulli N, Testa V, Capasso G, et al. Results of percutaneous longitudinal tenotomy for Achilles tendinopathy in middle- and long-distance runners. Am J Sports Med 1997;25(6):835–40.

24. Maffulli N, Longo U, Spiezia F, et al. Minimally invasive surgery for Achilles tendon pathologies. Open Access J Sports Med 2010;1:95–103.

25. Longo U, Ramamurthy C, Denaro V, et al. Minimally invasive stripping for chronic Achilles tendinopathy. Disabil Rehabil 2008;30(20–22):1709–13.

26. Steenstra F, van Dijk CN. Achilles tendoscopy. Foot Ankle Clin 2006;11(2):429–38, viii.

27. Maquirriain J. Surgical treatment of chronic achilles tendinopathy: long-term results of the endoscopic technique. J Foot Ankle Surg 2013;52(4):451–5.

28. Murphy GA. Surgical treatment of non-insertional Achilles tendinitis. Foot Ankle Clin 2009;14(4):651–61.

29. Elias I, Raikin S, Besser M, et al. Outcomes of chronic insertional Achilles tendinosis using FHL autograft through single incision. Foot Ankle Int 2009;30(3):197–204.

30. McGarvey W, Palumbo R, Baxter D, et al. Insertional Achilles tendinosis: surgical treatment through a central tendon splitting approach. Foot Ankle Int 2002;23(1):19–25.

31. Wagner E, Gould J, Kneidel M, et al. Technique and results of Achilles tendon detachment and reconstruction for insertional Achilles tendinosis. Foot Ankle Int 2006;27(9):677–84.

32. Georgiannos D, Kitridis D, Bisbinas I. Dorsal closing wedge calcaneal osteotomy for the treatment of Insertional Achilles Tendinopathy: A technical tip to optimize its results and reduce complications. Foot Ankle Surg 2018;24(2):115–8.

33. Nordio A, Chan J, Guzman J, et al. Percutaneous Zadek osteotomy for the treatment of insertional Achilles tendinopathy. Foot Ankle Surg; 2019.

34. Park YH, Kim TJ, Choi GW, et al. Achilles tendinosis does not always precede Achilles tendon rupture. Knee Surg Sports Traumatol Arthrosc 2018;27(10):3297–303.

35. Flik KR, Bush-Joseph CA, Bach BR Jr. Complete rupture of large tendons: risk factors, signs, and definitive treatment. Phys Sportsmed 2005;33(8):19–28.

36. Arner O, Lindholm A, Orell SR. Histologic changes in subcutaneous rupture of the Achilles tendon; a study of 74 cases. Acta Chir Scand 1959;116(5–6):484–90.

37. Movin T, Ryberg A, McBride D, et al. Acute rupture of the Achilles tendon. Foot Ankle Clin 2005;10(2):331–56.

38. Kauwe M. Acute Achilles Tendon Rupture. Clin Podiatr Med Surg 2017;34(2):229–43.

39. Christensen I. Rupture of the Achilles tendon; analysis of 57 cases. Acta Chir Scand 1953;106(1):50–60.

40. Maffulli N. The clinical diagnosis of subcutaneous tear of the Achilles tendon. A prospective study in 174 patients. Am J Sports Med 1998;26(2):266–70.
41. Simmonds FA. The diagnosis of the ruptured Achilles tendon. Practitioner 1957; 179(1069):56–8.
42. Thompson TC. A test for rupture of the tendo achillis. Acta Orthop Scand 1962; 32:461–5.
43. Scott BW, al Chalabi A. How the Simmonds-Thompson test works. J Bone Joint Surg Br 1992;74(2):314–5.
44. Matles AL. Rupture of the tendo achilles: another diagnostic sign. Bull Hosp Joint Dis 1975;36(1):48–51.
45. Reiman M, Burgi C, Strube E, et al. The utility of clinical measures for the diagnosis of achilles tendon injuries: a systematic review with meta-analysis. J Athl Train 2014;49(6):820–9.
46. Toygar O. Subkutane Ruptur Der Achillessehne (Diagnostik Und Behandlungsergebnisse). Helv Chir Acta 1947;14(3):209–31.
47. Dong Q, Fessell DP. Achilles tendon ultrasound technique. AJR Am J Roentgenol 2009;193(3):W173.
48. Longo U, Petrillo S, Maffulli N, et al. Acute achilles tendon rupture in athletes. Foot Ankle Clin 2013;18(2):319–38.
49. Schweitzer ME, Karasick D. MR imaging of disorders of the Achilles tendon. AJR Am J Roentgenol 2000;175(3):613–25.
50. Chiodo C, Glazebrook M, Bluman E, et al. Diagnosis and treatment of acute Achilles tendon rupture. J Am Acad Orthop Surg 2010;18(8):503–10.
51. Deng S, Sun Z, Zhang C, et al. Surgical Treatment Versus Conservative Management for Acute Achilles Tendon Rupture: A Systematic Review and Meta-Analysis of Randomized Controlled Trials. J Foot Ankle Surg 2017;56(6):1236–43.
52. Longo UG, Ronga M, Maffulli N. Acute ruptures of the achilles tendon. Sports Med Arthrosc Rev 2009;17(2):127–38.
53. Hsu A, Jones C, Cohen B, et al. Clinical Outcomes and Complications of Percutaneous Achilles Repair System Versus Open Technique for Acute Achilles Tendon Ruptures. Foot Ankle Int 2015;36(11):1279–86.
54. Ververidis A, Kalifis K, Touzopoulos P, et al. Percutaneous repair of the Achilles tendon rupture in athletic population. J Orthop 2016;13(1):57–61.
55. Braunstein M, Baumbach S, Boecker W, et al. Development of an accelerated functional rehabilitation protocol following minimal invasive Achilles tendon repair. Knee Surg Sports Traumatol Arthrosc 2018;26(3):846–53.
56. Aronow MS. Commentary on an article by Kevin Willits, MA, MD, FRCSC, et al.: "Operative versus nonoperative treatment of acute Achilles tendon ruptures: a multicenter randomized trial using accelerated functional rehabilitation". J Bone Joint Surg Am 2010;92(17):e32.
57. Renninger C, Kuhn K, Fellars T, et al. Operative and Nonoperative Management of Achilles Tendon Ruptures in Active Duty Military Population. Foot Ankle Int 2016; 37(3):269–73.
58. Soroceanu A, et al. Surgical versus nonsurgical treatment of acute Achilles tendon rupture: a meta-analysis of randomized trials. J Bone Joint Surg Am 2012;94(23):2136–43.
59. Trofa D, Miller J, Jang E, et al. Professional Athletes' Return to Play and Performance After Operative Repair of an Achilles Tendon Rupture. Am J Sports Med 2017;45(12): 2864–71.

60. Zellers JA, Carmont MR, Gravare Silbernagel K. Return to play post-Achilles tendon rupture: a systematic review and meta-analysis of rate and measures of return to play. Br J Sports Med 2016;50(21):1325–32.
61. Maffulli N, Longo U, Maffulli G, et al. Achilles tendon ruptures in elite athletes. Foot Ankle Int 2011;32(1):9–15.
62. Heikkinen J, Lantto I, Piilonen J, et al. Tendon Length, Calf Muscle Atrophy, and Strength Deficit After Acute Achilles Tendon Rupture: Long-Term Follow-up of Patients in a Previous Study. J Bone Joint Surg Am 2017;99(18):1509–15.
63. Rettig A, Liotta F, Klootwyk T, et al. Potential risk of rerupture in primary achilles tendon repair in athletes younger than 30 years of age. Am J Sports Med 2005;33(1):119–23.
64. Lerch T, Schwinghammer A, Schmaranzer F, et al. Return to Sport and Patient Satisfaction at 5-Year Follow-Up After Nonoperative Treatment for Acute Achilles Tendon Rupture. Foot Ankle Int 2020. [Epub ahead of print].

Osteochondral Defects of the Talus

How to Treat Without an Osteotomy

Matthew S. Conti, MD[a], J. Kent Ellington, MD, MS[b],
Steve B. Behrens, MD[a],*

KEYWORDS

- Osteochondral lesions of the talus • Microfracture
- Allograft cartilage extracellular matrix • Allograft juvenile hyaline cartilage
- Autologous chondrocyte implantation • Osteochondral autograft
- Ankle arthroscopy

KEY POINTS

- Appropriate surgical management of osteochondral lesions of the talus (OLTs) depends on size, location, and chronicity.
- Arthroscopic bone marrow stimulation techniques, such as microfracture, provide reliably good results for lesions less than 1 cm in diameter.
- Other techniques for smaller lesions include allograft cartilage extracellular matrix and allograft juvenile hyaline cartilage, which can be performed in a single stage using arthroscopy.
- Autologous chondrocyte implantation is a two-stage procedure indicated for defects greater than 1 cm^2. In the second stage, viable chondrocytes are implanted using either arthroscopy or an arthrotomy.
- For larger lesions with subchondral cysts, osteochondral autograft and allograft transplantation techniques can be used. These are typically performed through an arthrotomy; however, medial talar dome OLTs often require a medial malleolar osteotomy for access.

INTRODUCTION

Osteochondral lesions of the talus (OLTs) encompass a spectrum of articular cartilage and subchondral bone pathologic conditions that have a wide range of treatment options.[1-3] In the military population, the incidence of OLTs was found to be 27 per 100,000.[4] Proposed causes for OLTs include acute traumatic insult, repetitive chronic

[a] Hospital for Special Surgery, Weill Cornell Medical College, 535 East 70th Street, New York, NY 10021, USA; [b] OrthoCarolina Foot & Ankle Institute, 2001 Vail Avenue, Charlotte, NC 28207, USA
* Corresponding author.
E-mail address: behrenss@hss.edu

Clin Sports Med 39 (2020) 893–909
https://doi.org/10.1016/j.csm.2020.07.002
0278-5919/20/© 2020 Elsevier Inc. All rights reserved.

microtrauma to the ankle joint, and localized ischemia of the talus.[2,5] Recent literature suggests that location may not be a reliable predictor of the mechanism of injury.[6,7] Regardless of the cause, OLTs collectively demonstrate pathologic changes to the subchondral bone with or without involvement of the articular cartilage.[6] The natural history of these lesions is variable and not necessarily associated with eventual progression to osteoarthritis. In 1 study with an average follow-up of 21 years, only 2 of 30 patients with OLTs developed osteoarthritis, and only one of the 2 patients had severe symptoms.[8]

Diagnosis of OLTs begins with a comprehensive history and physical examination. Before advanced imaging, plain radiographs should be obtained in patients suspected of having an OLT. However, up to 50% of OLTs may not be visualized on radiographs alone.[9] MRI should be obtained to better evaluate OLTs, and in most cases, can be used to estimate the size of the lesion. In 1 retrospective study of 54 patients who underwent MRI of the ankle as well as an ankle arthroscopy, MRI correctly identified all OLTs in the cohort and all normal ankles.[10] After dividing the lesions into different grades based on the condition of the articular cartilage, MRI had a sensitivity of 95% and a specificity of 100% with a negative predictive value of 88% and a positive predictive value of 100%.[10] Further evaluation of OLTs may be performed using computed tomography (CT) scans, especially to evaluate subchondral bone and cystic changes. Although MRI can be used to estimate the size of the lesion, CT scans are more accurate for determining size and location of the lesion.[11] Diagnostic arthroscopy is not necessary to evaluate OLTs and has not been found to perform better than helical CT scans or MRI in the detection of OLTs.[9]

Management of OLTs depends on the size and stage of the lesion, patient activity level, and chronicity of the lesion. Nonoperative management is indicated for incidentally found lesions without clear clinical correlation of symptoms, minimally symptomatic patients with early-stage lesions and without loose intraarticular fragments, or patients who are improving clinically.[12] In a study of 48 patients with OLTs confirmed by MRI managed nonoperatively, 86% of ankles were pain free or had less pain at a minimum follow-up of 2 years.[12] Pain at final follow-up was correlated with depth of lesion on initial MRI and subchondral cyst formation at final follow-up MRI.[12] When nonoperative treatment is exhausted, surgical options should then be considered. Proper understanding of indications and potential complications for various techniques will enhance the surgeon's ability to select the most appropriate surgical procedure for each patient. Arthroscopic- and arthrotomy-based surgical techniques can be used in most cases of OLTs, thereby avoiding osteotomy for surgical treatment of these lesions.

SURGICAL MANAGEMENT

Surgical management of OLTs typically depends on the size and chronicity of the lesion. In general, acute large, detached osteochondral fragments may be directly repaired to the underlying bone.[13] Bone marrow stimulation using microfracture can be performed arthroscopically and has shown good clinical outcomes in lesions less than 15 mm in diameter.[1,2,14,15] For lesions not amenable to bone marrow stimulation techniques, other one-stage procedures, such as allograft cartilage extracellular matrix and allograft juvenile hyaline cartilage, have shown promising results.[16,17] Autologous chondrocyte implantation (ACI) is a two-stage procedure using chondrocytes cultured from the patient's healthy articular cartilage that has demonstrated good results in lesions greater than 1 cm^2.[18] Osteochondral autograft transplantation (OATS), in which hyaline cartilage from the knee is transplanted into the OLT, has been successfully used to treat lesions greater than 1.5 cm^2.[19–22] Other techniques, such as excision and curettage and osteochondral allografts, may also be used to treat OLTs.

Fixation

For large, loose osteochondral fragments, fixation of the lesion to the underlying bone is possible (**Fig. 1**).[3,13] Fixation is typically reserved for acute injuries with healthy-appearing articular cartilage attached to underlying bone and may be more prone to fail in chronic lesions with sclerotic borders.[13] One significant advantage of this technique is that it preserves the patient's native cartilage.[3] Options for fixation to the talus include Kirschner wires (K-wires), absorbable pins (eg, polylactic acid), headless screws, cortical bone pegs, or fibrin glue.[13,23,24]

Kumai and colleagues[24] used cortical bone pegs from the distal tibia to treat OLTs in 27 patients, including patients with unstable chronic lesions. For patients with sclerotic

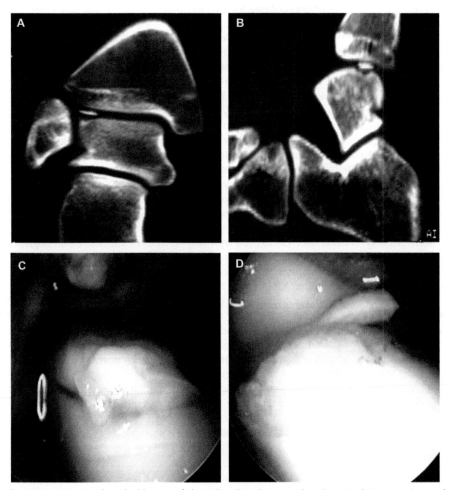

Fig. 1. Acute osteochondral lesion of the talus. (*A, B*) Coronal and sagittal CT scan views of an acute osteochondral lesion of the talus. (*C, D*) Arthroscopic images of the osteochondral lesion before fixation. (*Courtesy of* Martin J. O'Malley, M.D.)

subchondral beds, they performed concomitant subchondral drilling and then used 2 cortical pegs to anchor the fragment.[24] They reported good clinical outcomes in 24 of 27 ankles (89%) with no poor results and good radiologic improvement in 22 of 27 ankles (81%) at a mean follow-up of 7 years.[24] In a more recent study, Nakasa and colleagues[25] demonstrated good clinical and radiographic outcomes in 17 patients with OLTs treated with bioabsorbable pins. They divided patients into groups based on the preoperative bone condition of the lesion and found that good outcomes could be obtained at 1 year postoperatively when the bone quality of the fragment is poor as long as the articular cartilage surface was good.[25] On second-look arthroscopy in 15 patients, all OLTs demonstrated normal or near-normal cartilage.[25] Another study evaluated osteolytic changes following insertion of bioabsorbable pins for the treatment of talus osteochondral lesions.[26] On 1-year follow-up MRIs, 28.1% of the bioabsorbable pins had osteolytic changes around them.[26]

Excision and/or Curettage of Lesion

Excision alone or with chondroplasty for the treatment of OLTs has been used to address symptomatic lesions.[19,27] The partially detached lesion is removed, and there is no adjuvant treatment of the underlying defect. Indications for excision alone typically include small chronic OLTs with intact underlying subchondral bone. Success rates for excision alone are variable with reports ranging from 30% to 88%.[2] After excision, however, most OLTs are treated with some form of adjuvant therapy.[2]

In some cases, following excision of the lesion, curettage of the subchondral bone has been performed. A retrospective study by Robinson and colleagues[28] reviewing arthroscopic treatment of OLTs in 65 patients with a mean follow-up of 3.5 years suggested that excision and curettage of lesions had better outcomes than excision and microfracture. Excision and curettage led to good outcomes in 27 patients and poor outcomes in 5 patients, whereas excision and drilling led to good outcomes in 7 patients and poor outcomes 8 patients.[28] A systematic review of OLTs treated with excision and curettage led to a successful result in 77% of cases with individual studies citing good outcomes in 56% to 94% of patients, which is higher than what is reported for excision alone.[2]

Bone grafting has also been performed with varying rates of success as an adjuvant to curettage in patients with large subchondral cysts.[2,29,30] Kolker and colleagues[30] retrospectively looked at patient satisfaction and outcomes following curettage and autologous bone grafting for OLTs with a mean defect size of 12 mm × 15 mm. At an average follow-up of 37.4 months, they described 6 patients who failed treatment (46%) and required further surgery. Patient satisfaction was 46.2% in their study.[30] In contrast, Sawa and colleagues[29] performed autologous bone grafting from the distal tibia metaphysis for patients with OLTs and large subchondral cysts measuring, on average, 9 mm × 8.6 mm × 12.3 mm on preoperative CT scans. After lifting or removing the cartilage fragment to expose the underlying bone, the subchondral cyst was curetted and packed with autologous bone graft.[29] The cartilage fragment was then sutured back in place.[29] They reported significantly improved patient-reported outcomes at a minimum of 15-month follow-up, 100% patient satisfaction, and a decrease in the cyst size on plain radiographs.[29]

Bone Marrow Stimulation

Bone marrow stimulation using subchondral drilling with a K-wire or microfracture with an awl is usually performed after excision of the lesion and curettage of the calcified cartilage overlying the subchondral plate.[1–3,31] The subchondral plate is perforated at 3- to 4-mm intervals leading to a fibrin clot that contains growth factors and mesenchymal stem cells that stimulate healing with regenerative fibrocartilage.[32] The release of fatty droplets from the subchondral plate suggests that the appropriate drilling depth has been reached (**Fig. 2**).[1]

Indications for microfracture include symptomatic OLTs that are less than 15 mm in diameter because outcome data demonstrate higher failure rates for larger lesions.[1,2,14,15] Chuckpaiwong and colleagues[15] prospectively investigated the outcomes of microfracture in 105 patients with symptomatic OLTs with a mean follow-up of 31.5 months. In 73 patients with lesions less than 15 mm, they reported no failure of treatment; however, out of 32 patients with lesions larger than 15 mm, they had only 1 patient with a successful outcome.[15] The investigators concluded that microfracture for the surgical management of OLTs is appropriate for lesions less than 15 mm regardless of location.[15] Similarly, Choi and colleagues[33] retrospectively reviewed 120 ankles that underwent arthroscopic bone marrow stimulation of a symptomatic OLT. At mean follow-up of 44.5 months (range, 12–81 months), they showed clinical failure was 10.5% in ankles with a defect area less than 150 mm^2 (10 of 95 ankles), whereas ankles with a defect area greater than 150 mm^2 had a clinical failure of 80% (20 of 25 ankles).[33]

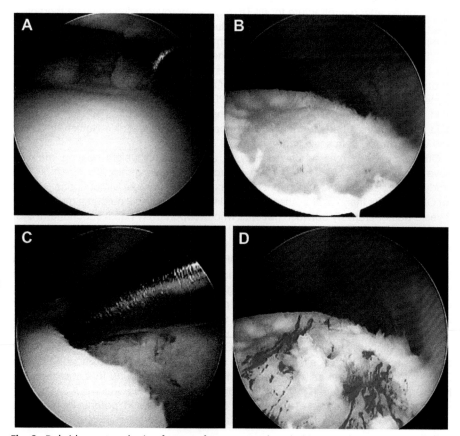

Fig. 2. Debridement and microfracture for an osteochondral lesion of the talus. (*A*) An osteochondral lesion with intact cartilage. (*B*) The lesion after debridement. (*C, D*) The microfracture technique with an awl. (*Courtesy of* Martin J. O'Malley, M.D.)

Short-term outcomes following microfracture for lesions less than 15 mm have generally been favorable.[1,2,34–36] Lee and colleagues[34] reported good to excellent outcomes following microfracture in 89% of 35 patients under the age of 50 years old with an OLT less than 15 mm^2 on MRI at a mean follow-up of 33 months. Becher and Thermann[36] reviewed 30 consecutive patients with cartilage defects of the talus and showed good to excellent outcomes in 83% of patients at a minimum follow-up of 22 months. In 3 patients who underwent subsequent arthroscopy for osteophyte removal, there was complete coverage of the OLTs with fibrocartilaginous tissue.[36]

Longer-term studies have demonstrated less encouraging results and suggest clinical outcomes deteriorate over time.[35,37] Polat and colleagues[35] reported that only 42.6% of patients who underwent microfracture for an average defect size of 1.7 cm^2 described no symptoms at a minimum of 5-year follow-up. Thirty-three percent of patients in their study had a one-stage increase in their arthritis grade on final radiographic follow-up.[35] A more recent study looked at subchondral bone marrow edema on MRIs in 52 patients who underwent microfracture for OLTs less than 15 mm or 150 mm^2 without a large cystic component.[38] Seventy-four patients had subchondral bone marrow edema at 4-year follow-up, and those patients with subchondral bone marrow edema had worse clinical outcomes than the patients without evidence of bone marrow edema.[38]

Outcomes after microfracture for OLTs may be improved using adjuvant therapies, such as platelet-rich plasma (PRP) and hyaluronic acid.[22,39,40] One randomized trial compared microfracture surgery alone with microfracture and PRP for the treatment of OLTs less than 20 mm in diameter, and the investigators reported that patients in the PRP group had better clinical outcomes at a mean follow-up of 16 months.[22] Another study randomized 40 patients with OLTs less than 15 mm^2 to microfracture alone (control group), microfracture with PRP, and microfracture with hyaluronic acid.[39] At a minimum follow-up of 11 months, patients who had PRP or hyaluronic acid adjuvants had better American Orthopaedic Foot and Ankle Society (AOFAS) and visual analog pain scale scores than the control group.[39]

Other factors, such as subchondral cysts, age, and early weight-bearing, may not have significant effects on postoperative outcomes following microfracture.[41–43] In a study of 102 patients who underwent arthroscopic microfracture without bone grafting for OLTs smaller than 20 mm^2, there was no difference in clinical outcome measures at 2 years postoperatively between patients who preoperatively had a subchondral cyst identified by MRI and those who did not.[41] Another study found that increasing age was not an independent risk factor for a poor outcome after microfracture for an OLT at a minimum of 2 years postoperatively.[42] A prospective, randomized controlled trial allocated 81 ankles treated with arthroscopic microfracture to either delayed weight-bearing, which consisted of keeping patients non-weight-bearing for 6 weeks, or early weight-bearing, which consisted of partial weight-bearing in a walking boot for 2 weeks followed by full weight-bearing as soon as tolerated afterward.[43] There were no differences in patient-reported outcome scores at a minimum of 2-year follow-up.[43]

Subchondral drilling for the treatment of OLTs also relies on recruiting bone marrow elements to repair cartilage lesions.[2,3,44] In an animal-model study comparing microfracture to subchondral drilling in rabbits, the investigators found that microfracture holes can become impeded by fractured bone around the holes, which potentially prevents viable bone marrow element from being released and potentially inhibiting repair.[44] They did not find that subchondral drilling led to substantial heat necrosis in their models.[44]

Subchondral drilling can be performed through either antegrade (transmalleolar) or retrograde approaches. Retrograde approaches are most commonly used when the articular cartilage overlying the lesion is intact with a concomitant subchondral cyst.[13,45,46] Retrograde drilling can be performed through a sinus tarsi approach for medial OLTs or through a posterolateral approach.[45,46] Kono and colleagues[45] retrospectively reviewed 30 patients who underwent either antegrade transmalleolar drilling (n = 19) or retrograde drilling through a posterolateral approach (n = 11). On 1-year postoperative MRIs, they found that 57.9% of lesions were unchanged in the transmalleolar group compared with 72.8% in the retrograde drilling group.[45] In a systematic review of retrograde drilling for OLTs, 88% of patients were reported to have a successful outcome.[2] A retrospective study by Choi and Lee[31] of 90 ankles with OLTs less than 20 mm^2 treated with either antegrade subchondral drilling or microfracture found no differences in clinical outcome scores with a minimum follow-up of 2 years.

Allograft Cartilage Extracellular Matrix, Allograft Juvenile Hyaline Cartilage, and Minced Autograft Cartilage

Allograft cartilage extracellular matrix and allograft juvenile hyaline cartilage have both been reported to treat OLT.[16,17,47] Minced autograft cartilage has been used in the treatment of osteochondral lesions at other sites but has not been reported in the talus.[48] One of the advantages of these techniques is that they can be performed arthroscopically in a single stage.

Allograft cartilage matrix consists of type II collagen, proteoglycans, and cartilaginous growth fractures that are found in normal hyaline cartilage, and when applied to OLTs at the microfracture site, the allograft cartilage matrix serves as a scaffold with which marrow elements can interact.[16] Few studies have reported the results of allograft cartilage matrix for the treatment of OLTs.[16] Ahmad and Maltenfort[16] reported the results of microfracture and allograft extracellular matrix in 30 patients with OLTs of 15 mm^2 or smaller. At a minimum follow-up of 12 months, the investigators reported good or excellent patient satisfaction in 27 patients (90%).[16] Complications in 4 patients included a deep vein thrombosis in 1 patient, incomplete chondral healing of their OLT on 6-month postoperative CT scans in 2 patients, and the development of symptomatic ankle arthritis 19 months after surgery in 1 patient.[16]

Allograft juvenile cartilage is a cartilaginous tissue graft from donors under 13 years old and is designed to fill the OLT with hyaline-line cartilage (**Fig. 3**).[3,47] The largest

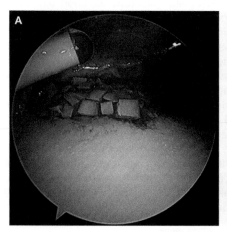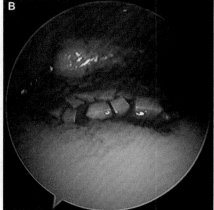

Fig. 3. (*A, B*) Osteochondral lesion of the talus repaired with particulated juvenile cartilage and fibrin glue. (*Courtesy of* Martin J. O'Malley, M.D.)

cohort of patients was reported by Coetzee and colleagues.[17] In this multicenter study, 24 ankles were enrolled with an OLT size between 50 and 300 mm^2 and a minimum follow-up of 12 months.[17] Seventy-eight percent of ankles demonstrated good to excellent clinical outcome scores, and they described 1 partial graft delamination that occurred at 16 months postoperatively.[17] In lesions between 10 and 15 mm, 92% had good to excellent results.[17] More recently, Dekker and colleagues[49] reported their results of particulated juvenile cartilage allograft transplantation in 15 patients with OLTs between 66 and 299 mm^2 and a minimum of 12-month follow-up. Male patients and patients with lesions greater than 125 mm^2 were at higher risk of treatment failure.[49] They reported a failure rate of 40% in their study with half of the failure patients requiring a subsequent cartilage procedure and the other half of the failure patients reporting no improvement in their pain after the procedure.[49]

Autologous and Matrix-Based Chondrocyte Implantation

ACI is a two-stage procedure indicated for full-thickness, large (>1 cm^2) OLTs that attempts to regenerate tissue with biomechanical properties similar to normal hyaline cartilage.[2,3,18] In the first stage, a biopsy of viable chondrocytes is taken from areas of normal articular cartilage, such as the margin of the distal tibia or talus or the femoral intercondylar notch.[18,50–53] Some investigators have argued against using articular cartilage from the ankle joint because small changes in the cartilage surface of the distal tibia and talus may impair the mechanics of the joint.[50] Chondrocytes from the biopsy are then cultured over the subsequent 2 to 6 weeks before the second stage of the procedure.[3] In the second stage, most talar ACI procedures are performed using a scaffold such as a type I/III bilayer collagen membrane (matrix-induced chondrocyte implantation, MACI) in order to hold the implanted cells in place during the second stage of the procedure.[1,3,54] Another technique using a periosteum patch instead of a scaffold is more technically demanding and has significant limitations.[3] Weight-bearing is typically restricted postoperatively, but early gentle range-of-motion exercises are begun soon after surgery in order to prevent chondrocyte atrophy.[50] MRI using T2 mapping at an average of 5 years follow-up after ACI demonstrated normal-appearing hyaline cartilage covering a mean 69% of the repaired OLT area with fibrocartilaginous tissue covering, on average, another 17%.[55]

Outcomes following ACI have been reported in multiple case series and have been consistently good.[18,51–53,56] Whittaker and colleagues[56] first reported short-term outcomes at a minimum of 12 months following ACI for treatment of OLTs. They included 10 patients with OLTs ranging from 1 to 4 cm^2 based on intraoperative examination.[56] One-year postoperative repeat ankle arthroscopy demonstrated that the defects in all patients were filled.[56] Nine of out 10 patients stated that they were "pleased" or "extremely pleased" after surgery, and 1 patient was no better.[56]

In a longer-term study, Kwak and colleagues[53] reviewed 29 consecutive patients who underwent ACI after failing previous drilling and/or microfracture for OLTs with a mean size of 198 mm^2 (range, 80–500 mm^2). Follow-up was at a minimum of 24 months and a mean of 70 months (range, 24–129 months). The investigators used a periosteal graft as a scaffold for the cultured chondrocytes and applied fibrin glue to the final defect.[53] For large cysts, they used autologous bone grafting to fill the defect and then placed the periosteal graft on top of the bone graft.[53] Patients were kept non-weight-bearing for 2 weeks and then began touchdown weight-bearing until 6 weeks when they were made full weight-bearing.[53] At final follow-up, 90% of patients were satisfied with their procedure.[53] There was no correlation between lesion size and postoperative AOFAS score.[53] On second-look arthroscopy in 25 patients at a mean of 16 months, there was no exposed bone in any patients, and on postoperative MRIs at a mean of 65 months, 22 of 24 patients had good fill of the repair site.[53]

Anders and colleagues[51] reported their results of MACI using a porcine collagen type I/III scaffold in 22 consecutive patients with OLTs greater than 1.0 cm^2 and a minimum of 3-year follow-up. They noted sustained improvements in clinical outcome scores from preoperatively to 5 years postoperatively.[51] Giannini and colleagues[52] studied 46 patients with a mean OLT size of 1.6 cm^2 treated with ACI. At an average follow-up of 87.2 months, they reported significant improvement in clinical outcome scores with only 3 failures in their group, which had to undergo revision surgery.[52] All 4 professional soccer players in their study were able to resume their previous level of activity.[52] These results suggest consistently good longer-term outcomes following ACI procedures for OLTs. However, ACI is expensive compared with bone marrow stimulation techniques, and it is not clear whether ACI has better long-term outcomes than microfracture or drilling especially for lesions between 1.0 and 1.5 cm^2.[2,3]

Osteochondral Autograft Transplantation

OATS is a single-step surgical procedure performed by harvesting one or many (mosaicplasty) bone-hyaline cartilage plugs from the knee and subsequently transplanting them into the talar lesion (**Fig. 4**).[3,57] OATS is indicated for larger lesions, typically greater than 1.5 cm^2, highly cystic lesions, or lesions that have failed debridement and microfracture.[1,3] Treatment of OLTs with OATS must weigh the opportunity to improve upon the high failure rates of microfracture for larger lesions with the additional complications and more demanding technical aspects of OATS.[1] However, it can be challenging to perform this procedure without medial malleolar because implantation requires a perpendicular approach to the OLT.

A significant limitation of OATS is donor site morbidity.[57,58] Paul and colleagues[57] followed 112 patients who were treated using an OATS procedure using graft obtained from an asymptomatic knee for an OLT for a minimum of 2 years. Patients' satisfaction with their donor knee was the best predictor of postoperative functional outcomes.[57] Functional outcomes were not affected by the age of the patient, size of the donor graft, or number of donor grafts harvested.[57] In another study that examined donor site morbidity after mosaicplasties with grafts harvest from an asymptomatic knee to treat OLTs, Reddy and colleagues[58] looked at 11 patients with a mean follow-up of 47 months and found that patients with lower functional outcome scores reported knee instability in daily activities as the most common issue. One patient required a tibial tubercle osteotomy and lateral retinacular release to address subsequent knee pain and patella instability after the mosaicplasty.[58]

Outcomes following OATS have been consistently good with success rates between 74% and 100%.[2] Gobbi and colleagues[19] assigned 32 patients to chondroplasty, microfracture, or OATS, and at a minimum of 2 years follow-up, found no difference in patient-reported outcomes between the groups. However, they did report better outcomes were associated with smaller lesions in the microfracture and OATS groups.[19] Paul and colleagues[20] retrospectively reviewed 131 patients with a minimum follow-up of 2 years who underwent OATS for treatment of a symptomatic OLT. The frequency and duration of sports activity did not change significantly after surgery, and they reported that 71% of their patients were very satisfied or satisfied after surgery.[20] Woelfle and colleagues[59] also found good clinical results at a minimum of 14 months' follow-up and did not find that more than 1 osteochondral graft, body mass index greater than 25, or failed previous surgery affected outcomes. The same group noted that patients older than 40 years at the time of surgery had lower Hospital for Special Surgery patella scores than younger patients, which suggests

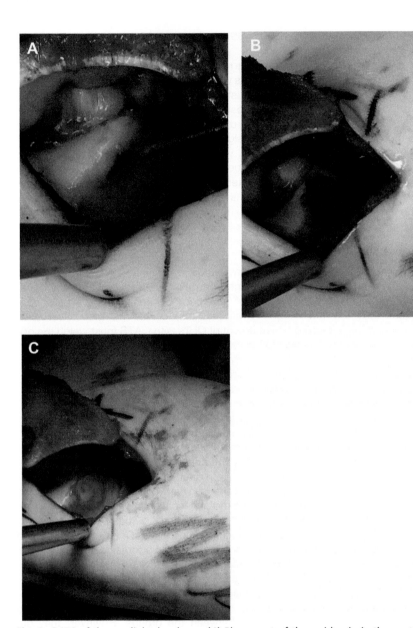

Fig. 4. OATS of the medial talar dome. (*A*) Placement of the guide pin in the center of the lesion before using the cannulated reamer. (*B, C*) The osteochondral plug is placed in the resultant defect. This image demonstrates placement of an OATS plug in the medial talar dome. For access to this lesion, a medial malleolar osteotomy was required. (*Courtesy of* Martin J. O'Malley, M.D.)

an increase in donor-site morbidity in older patients.[21] Guney and colleagues[37] performed a nonrandomized trial to compare mosaicplasty to arthroscopic microfracture with and without PRP in 54 patients with OLTs. They did not describe lesion size in the groups; follow-up was significantly shorter in the mosaicplasty (mean 30.1 months compared with 47.3 months in the microfracture group alone), and patients in the mosaicplasty group had significantly higher baseline preoperative pain scores.[37] Post-operatively, patients in the mosaicplasty group had a more significant change in their pain scores than other groups, but this may have been confounded by the shorter follow-up and higher baseline preoperative pain score.[37] Five patients in the microfracture surgery group required reoperation because of worsening pain, and no other complications were noted.[37]

Osteochondral Allograft

Osteochondral allograft transplantation uses viable articular cartilage and subchondral bone from cadaver graft that can be matched to a specified size and orientation of curvature of the talus.[60] Indications include large OLTs greater than 1.5 cm^2 and are similar to those for OATS.[60] A CT scan of the patient's contralateral talus can be used as a template in order to match the appropriate-sized allograft graft.[60] The benefits of avoiding donor-site morbidity must be weighed against the risks inherent to allografts, such as disease transmission and allograft rejection, although these are rare.[60] One study investigated 40 patients who had recurrent OLTs after failing arthroscopic treatment or a primary OLT larger than 1.5 cm^2 and were randomized to either OATS or osteochondral allograft.[61] At a minimum of 12 months of follow-up, the investigators reported similar postoperative outcomes but lower rates of healing in the allograft group.[61]

Osteochondral allografts have had variable results.[62–64] Raikin[62] prospectively followed 15 patients with symptomatic OLTs with an average lesion volume of 6059 mm^3 treated with a fresh osteochondral allograft and had a minimum follow-up of 2 years postoperatively. Clinical outcome scores were improved at final follow-up, and 11 of the patients had good or excellent results.[62] Two patients subsequently underwent ankle arthrodesis at 32 and 76 months.[62] In another study that retrospectively reviewed 16 patients who underwent a fresh osteochondral allograft transplantation for OLTs and had an average duration of follow-up of 4.1 years, 10 patients reported a good or excellent result with persistent pain in 6 patients.[63] The investigators reported that 5 ankles were considered failures.[63] Although osteochondral allografts avoid donor-site morbidity, their higher failure rates compared with OATS suggest that their indications should be limited to salvage procedures or for patients seeking to delay more definitive operations, such as total ankle replacement or ankle arthrodesis.

Talus Replacement

In patients with large cystic OLTs that have failed prior procedures, a hemi-talus or total talus may be used as a salvage procedure. In a recent case series of 15 patients with avascular necrosis of the talus who were treated with custom 3-dimensionally printed total talar replacements, the investigators reported significant improvements in clinical outcome scores postoperatively and a decrease in postoperative pain scores at 1-year follow-up.[65] They concluded that total talus replacement is an option for talar avascular necrosis.[65] However, these same principles may apply in patients with large OLTs who have failed previous surgical management.

TECHNIQUES WITHOUT AN OSTEOTOMY

Many OLTs can be addressed without requiring an osteotomy. Anterior and posterior ankle arthroscopic techniques are commonly used with good or excellent results.[66] Extension of the arthroscopic portals or formal arthrotomies may be required to insert large grafts. The surgical approach and procedure should be based on characteristics of the lesion. The location of the lesion on the talar dome influences the approach used.[67] Additional considerations for surgical technique include the size and stability of the lesion, chronicity of the lesion, subchondral bone cysts, and failure of previous surgery.

Arthroscopy

Anterior and posterior arthroscopy can be used to access almost the entirety of the talar dome.[67] Anterior arthroscopy is performed with the patient lying supine on the operating room table with a tourniquet applied to the ipsilateral thigh. The patient's foot is brought to the edge of the operating room table and a well-padded thigh holder can be secured underneath the patient's posterior thigh to elevate the foot. After prepping and draping the patient, a noninvasive ankle distractor can be applied to the patient's foot, which can be attached to a device mounted on the operating room table or to a sterile strap placed around the waist of the surgeon. Alternatively, dorsiflexion of the foot may be used by the surgeon by leaning against the patient's foot at the edge of the bed.

Anterior arthroscopy uses an anteromedial and anterolateral as the primary portals. The anteromedial portal is the primary viewing portal and is located just medial to the tibialis anterior tendon at the level of the ankle joint. This portal is established first, and some surgeons choose to use a needle on a syringe to identify the trajectory of the portal and inject normal saline into the joint. Care is taken to avoid the saphenous neurovascular structures using a nick-and-spread technique in which the skin is incised using a 15-blade scalpel followed by a small clamp to spread through the soft tissues and enter the joint.[68] A 30° angle 2.7-mm arthroscope is then inserted into the joint. The anterolateral portal is made lateral to the peroneus tertius tendon under direct visualization with care to avoid the dorsal intermediate cutaneous branch of the superficial peroneal nerve. Traction on the fourth toe may help the surgeon identify this branch of the superficial peroneal nerve. The nick-and-spread technique is again used to avoid damaging nearby neurovascular structures. Noninvasive traction with up to 30° of plantarflexion or dorsiflexion may help to improve the area of visualization of the talus.[67,68] One study reported that anterior arthroscopy was significantly better than posterior arthroscopy for visualizing central lesions of the talus with anterior arthroscopy being able to access 87.7% of the central one-third of the talar dome compared with 74.3% when using posterior arthroscopy.[67] In that same study, anterior arthroscopy is able to visualize 58.6% of the talar dome and 100% of the anterior one-third of the talar dome.[67]

Posterior arthroscopy requires that the patient is placed in the prone position with the ankle off the edge of the bed or with a triangular cushion underneath the distal tibia.[69] Two portals are again used. The primary viewing portal is the posterolateral portal, which is located between the peroneal and Achilles tendons at the level of the distal tip of the lateral malleolus. The nick-and-spread technique is used to avoid injury to the sural nerve. The posteromedial portal is subsequently created with care to avoid injuring the neurovascular bundle that lies medial to the flexor hallucis longus tendon. Posterior arthroscopy allows visualization of 49.8% of the talar dome and may be improved with ankle distraction.[67]

Arthroscopy alone may be used to treat smaller lesions often without significant cystic components. Excision and debridement of OLTs may be performed arthroscopically using a 4.5-mm or 5.5-mm shaver.[68] Antegrade transmalleolar and retrograde drilling using a K-wire is done in conjunction with ankle arthroscopy in order to visualize the lesion. Similarly, OLTs amenable to microfracture are typically treated using ankle arthroscopy, which can reliably access most sites on the talar dome.[67]

Allograft cartilage extracellular matrix, allograft juvenile hyaline cartilage, and minced autograft cartilage can be inserted through a cannula arthroscopically in a single stage. However, depending on the size and location of the lesion, these techniques occasionally require an arthrotomy. In addition, the inability to use fluid during the implantation stage can make visualization difficult when compared with an open approach.

Arthrotomy

An ankle arthrotomy may be necessary to address larger or cystic OLTs. Indications include fixation of acute lesions, ACI, OATS, osteochondral allograft transplantation, or talus replacement. Lateral and more anterior lesions are easier to visualize using an arthrotomy than medial lesions because of the medial malleolus. Plantarflexion of the ankle can provide increased visualization of the talar dome and is especially useful for laterally based lesions where an osteotomy is often unnecessary. Releasing the lateral ligaments (anterior talofibular and calcaneofibular ligaments) can improve visualization for lateral talar dome lesions.

   Although an articular cartilage biopsy as part of an ACI procedure is typically performed arthroscopically, the second stage may be performed using either arthroscopy or an arthrotomy.[51,55] After removing saline from the joint, the scaffold and cells can be inserted into the dry ankle joint through a cannula and applied to the lesion using a probe.[55] OATS and osteochondral allograft transplantation may require larger incisions to insert the graft. Lateral and anterior talar dome lesions can be accessed through an arthrotomy and plantarflexion. Temporary invasive distraction has been proposed as a technique to improve visualization of lateral OLTs with few complications.[70] However, a medial malleolar osteotomy is typically required to adequately expose central and posterior medial talar dome lesions when performing OATS.[71] Finally, talus replacement for severe OLTs with significant bone loss or avascular necrosis of the talus may be performed through a direct anterior arthrotomy of the ankle.[65]

SUMMARY

OLTs encompass a diverse group of pathologic conditions affecting both articular cartilage and subchondral bone. Initial evaluation of the lesion includes standard radiographs of the ankle and an MRI. CT scans are useful as an adjunct to MRI in the evaluation of subchondral cysts. For patients who have failed nonoperative management, surgical treatment is indicated and depends on the size, location, and chronicity of the lesion. Lesions less than 1 cm in diameter are associated with better outcomes and are amenable to arthroscopically assisted bone marrow stimulation techniques, such as microfracture or subchondral drilling. Allograft cartilage extracellular matrix and allograft juvenile hyaline cartilage may also be used for smaller lesions and can be inserted through an arthroscopic cannula in a single stage. ACI is indicated for lesions larger than 1 cm^2 but requires 2 stages. Arthroscopy or arthrotomy may be used for the second-stage implantation. For large OLTs associated with or without bone loss, osteochondral autograft or allograft transplantation may be performed. An arthrotomy is used in these techniques to insert the graft. When using OATS or osteochondral allograft transplantation for medial talar dome lesions, arthrotomy alone does not provide adequate access, and a medial malleolar osteotomy is frequently required.

DISCLOSURE

M. S. Conti: This author has nothing to disclose. J.K. Ellington: Amniox: paid consultant; Arthrex: IP royalties; Kinos: stock or stock options; Medline: IP royalties, paid consultant, paid presenter or speaker; Medshape: stock or stock options; Nuvasive: paid consultant; Synthes: IP royalties, paid consultant, paid presenter or speaker; Wright Medical Technology: paid consultant. S.B. Behrens: This author has nothing to disclose.

REFERENCES

1. Murawski CD, Kennedy JG. Operative treatment of osteochondral lesions of the talus. J Bone Joint Surg 2013;95(11):1045–54.
2. Zengerink M, Struijs PAA, Tol JL, et al. Treatment of osteochondral lesions of the talus: a systematic review. Knee Surg Sports Traumatol Arthrosc 2010;18(2): 238–46.
3. Kraeutler MJ, Chahla J, Dean CS, et al. Current concepts review update: osteochondral lesions of the talus. Foot Ankle Int 2017;38(3):331–42.
4. Orr JD, Dawson LK, Garcia EJ, et al. Incidence of osteochondral lesions of the talus in the United States military. Foot Ankle Int 2011;32(10):948–54.
5. O'Loughlin PF, Heyworth BE, Kennedy JG. Current concepts in the diagnosis and treatment of osteochondral lesions of the ankle. Am J Sports Med 2010;38(2): 392–404.
6. Raikin SM, Elias I, Zoga AC, et al. Osteochondral lesions of the talus: localization and morphologic data from 424 patients using a novel anatomical grid scheme. Foot Ankle Int 2007;28(2):154–61.
7. Orr JD, Dutton JR, Fowler JT. Anatomic location and morphology of symptomatic, operatively treated osteochondral lesions of the talus. Foot Ankle Int 2012;33(12): 1051–7.
8. Bauer M, Jonsson K, Lindén B. Osteochondritis dissecans of the ankle. A 20-year follow-up study. J Bone Joint Surg Br 1987;69(1):93–6.
9. Verhagen RAW, Maas M, Dijkgraaf MGW, et al. Prospective study on diagnostic strategies in osteochondral lesions of the talus. Is MRI superior to helical CT? J Bone Joint Surg Br 2005;87(1):41–6.
10. Mintz DN, Tashjian GS, Connell DA, et al. Osteochondral lesions of the talus: a new magnetic resonance grading system with arthroscopic correlation. Arthroscopy 2003;19(4):353–9.
11. Watson TS, Shurnas PS, Denker J. Diagnosis, physical exam, and imaging for osteochondral lesions of the talus. Foot Ankle Orthop 2018;3(3). 2473011418S0026.
12. Klammer G, Maquieira GJ, Spahn S, et al. Natural history of nonoperatively treated osteochondral lesions of the talus. Foot Ankle Int 2015;36(1):24–31.
13. Badekas T, Takvorian M, Souras N. Treatment principles for osteochondral lesions in foot and ankle. Int Orthop 2013;37(9):1697–706.
14. Cuttica DJ, Smith WB, Hyer CF, et al. Osteochondral lesions of the talus: predictors of clinical outcome. Foot Ankle Int 2011;32(11):1045–51.
15. Chuckpaiwong B, Berkson EM, Theodore GH. Microfracture for osteochondral lesions of the ankle: outcome analysis and outcome predictors of 105 cases. Arthroscopy 2008;24(1):106–12.
16. Ahmad J, Maltenfort M. Arthroscopic treatment of osteochondral lesions of the talus with allograft cartilage matrix. Foot Ankle Int 2017;38(8):855–62.
17. Coetzee JC, Giza E, Schon LC, et al. Treatment of osteochondral lesions of the talus with particulated juvenile cartilage. Foot Ankle Int 2013;34(9):1205–11.
18. Buda R, Vannini F, Castagnini F, et al. Regenerative treatment in osteochondral lesions of the talus: autologous chondrocyte implantation versus one-step bone marrow derived cells transplantation. Int Orthop 2015;39(5):893–900.

19. Gobbi A, Francisco RA, Lubowitz JH, et al. Osteochondral lesions of the talus: randomized controlled trial comparing chondroplasty, microfracture, and osteochondral autograft transplantation. Arthroscopy 2006;22(10):1085–92.
20. Paul J, Sagstetter M, Lämmle L, et al. Sports activity after osteochondral transplantation of the talus. Am J Sports Med 2012;40(4):870–4.
21. Woelfle JV, Reichel H, Nelitz M. Indications and limitations of osteochondral autologous transplantation in osteochondritis dissecans of the talus. Knee Surg Sports Traumatol Arthrosc 2013;21(8):1925–30.
22. Guney A, Akar M, Karaman I, et al. Clinical outcomes of platelet rich plasma (PRP) as an adjunct to microfracture surgery in osteochondral lesions of the talus. Knee Surg Sports Traumatol Arthrosc 2015;23(8):2384–9.
23. Nakagawa S, Hara K, Minami G, et al. Arthroscopic fixation technique for osteochondral lesions of the talus. Foot Ankle Int 2010;31(11):1025–7.
24. Kumai T, Takakura Y, Kitada C, et al. Fixation of osteochondral lesions of the talus using cortical bone pegs. J Bone Joint Surg Br 2002;84(3):369–74.
25. Nakasa T, Ikuta Y, Ota Y, et al. Clinical results of bioabsorbable pin fixation relative to the bone condition for osteochondral lesion of the talus. Foot Ankle Int 2019; 40(12):1388–96.
26. Nakasa T, Ikuta Y, Tsuyuguchi Y, et al. MRI tracking of the effect of bioabsorbable pins on bone marrow edema after fixation of the osteochondral fragment in the talus. Foot Ankle Int 2019;40(3):323–9.
27. Kelbérine F, Frank A. Arthroscopic treatment of osteochondral lesions of the talar dome: a retrospective study of 48 cases. Arthroscopy 1994;15(1):77–84.
28. Robinson DE, Winson IG, Harries WJ, et al. Arthroscopic treatment of osteochondral lesions of the talus. J Bone Joint Surg Br 2003;85(7):989–93.
29. Sawa M, Nakasa T, Ikuta Y, et al. Outcome of autologous bone grafting with preservation of articular cartilage to treat osteochondral lesions of the talus with large associated subchondral cysts. J Bone Joint Surg Am 2018;100B(5):590–5.
30. Kolker D, Murray M, Wilson M. Osteochondral defects of the talus treated with autologous bone grafting. J Bone Joint Surg Br 2004;86(4):521–6.
31. Choi JI, Lee KB. Comparison of clinical outcomes between arthroscopic subchondral drilling and microfracture for osteochondral lesions of the talus. Knee Surg Sports Traumatol Arthrosc 2016;24(7):2140–7.
32. Min BH, Choi WH, Lee YS, et al. Effect of different bone marrow stimulation techniques (BSTs) on MSCs mobilization. J Orthop Res 2013;31(11):1814–9.
33. Choi WJ, Park KK, Kim BS, et al. Osteochondral lesion of the talus: is there a critical defect size for poor outcome? Am J Sports Med 2009;37(10):1974–80.
34. Lee KB, Bai L Bin, Chung JY, et al. Arthroscopic microfracture for osteochondral lesions of the talus. Knee Surg Sports Traumatol Arthrosc 2010;18(2):247–53.
35. Polat G, Erşen A, Erdil ME, et al. Long-term results of microfracture in the treatment of talus osteochondral lesions. Knee Surg Sports Traumatol Arthrosc 2016;24(4):1299–303.
36. Becher C, Thermann H. Results of microfracture in the treatment of articular cartilage defects of the talus. Foot Ankle Int 2005;26(8):583–9.
37. Guney A, Yurdakul E, Karaman I, et al. Medium-term outcomes of mosaicplasty versus arthroscopic microfracture with or without platelet-rich plasma in the treatment of osteochondral lesions of the talus. Knee Surg Sports Traumatol Arthrosc 2016;24(4):1293–8.
38. Shimozono Y, Hurley ET, Yasui Y, et al. The presence and degree of bone marrow edema influence midterm clinical outcomes after microfracture for osteochondral lesions of the talus. Am J Sports Med 2018;46(10):2503–8.

39. Görmeli G, Karakaplan M, Görmeli CA, et al. Clinical effects of platelet-rich plasma and hyaluronic acid as an additional therapy for talar osteochondral lesions treated with microfracture surgery. Foot Ankle Int 2015;36(8):891–900.
40. Doral MN, Bilge O, Batmaz G, et al. Treatment of osteochondral lesions of the talus with microfracture technique and postoperative hyaluronan injection. Knee Surg Sports Traumatol Arthrosc 2012;20(7):1398–403.
41. Lee KB, Park HW, Cho HJ, et al. Comparison of arthroscopic microfracture for osteochondral lesions of the talus with and without subchondral cyst. Am J Sports Med 2015;43(8):1951–6.
42. Choi WJ, Kim BS, Lee JW. Osteochondral lesion of the talus: could age be an indication for arthroscopic treatment? Am J Sports Med 2012;40(2):419–24.
43. Lee DH, Lee KB, Jung ST, et al. Comparison of early versus delayed weightbearing outcomes after microfracture for small to midsized osteochondral lesions of the talus. Am J Sports Med 2012;40(9):2023–8.
44. Chen H, Sun J, Hoemann CD, et al. Drilling and microfracture lead to different bone structure and necrosis during bone-marrow stimulation for cartilage repair. J Orthop Res 2009;27(11):1432–8.
45. Kono M, Takao M, Naito K, et al. Retrograde drilling for osteochondral lesions of the talar dome. Am J Sports Med 2006;34(9):1450–6.
46. Berlet GC, Berlet GC, Philbin TM, et al. Retrograde drilling of osteochondral lesions of the talus. Foot Ankle Spec 2008;1(4):207–9.
47. Cerrato R. Particulated juvenile articular cartilage allograft transplantation for osteochondral lesions of the talus. Foot Ankle Clin 2019;18(1):79–87.
48. Levinson C, Cavalli E, Sindi DM, et al. Chondrocytes from device-minced articular cartilage show potent outgrowth into fibrin and collagen hydrogels. Orthop J Sports Med 2019;7(9). 2325967119867761.
49. Dekker TJ, Steele JR, Federer AE, et al. Efficacy of particulated juvenile cartilage allograft transplantation for osteochondral lesions of the talus. Foot Ankle Int 2018;39(3):278–83.
50. Mandelbaum BR, Gerhardt MB, Peterson L. Autologous chondrocyte implantation of the talus. Arthroscopy 2003;19(10 SUPPL. 1):129–37.
51. Anders S, Goetz J, Schubert T, et al. Treatment of deep articular talus lesions by matrix associated autologous chondrocyte implantation - results at five years. Int Orthop 2012;36(11):2279–85.
52. Giannini S, Buda R, Ruffilli A, et al. Arthroscopic autologous chondrocyte implantation in the ankle joint. Knee Surg Sports Traumatol Arthrosc 2014;22(6):1311–9.
53. Kwak SK, Kern BS, Ferkel RD, et al. Autologous chondrocyte implantation of the ankle: 2- to 10-year results. Am J Sports Med 2014;42(9):2156–64.
54. Gomoll AH, Probst C, Farr J, et al. Use of a type I/III bilayer collagen membrane decreases reoperation rates for symptomatic hypertrophy after autologous chondrocyte implantation. Am J Sports Med 2009;37(1_suppl):20S–3S.
55. Battaglia M, Vannini F, Buda R, et al. Arthroscopic autologous chondrocyte implantation in osteochondral lesions of the talus: mid-term T2-mapping MRI evaluation. Knee Surg Sports Traumatol Arthrosc 2011;19(8):1376–84.
56. Whittaker JP, Smith G, Makwana N, et al. Early results of autologous chondrocyte implantation in the talus. J Bone Joint Surg Br 2005;87(2):179–83.
57. Paul J, Sagstetter A, Kriner M, et al. Donor-site morbidity after osteochondral autologous transplantation for lesions of the talus. J Bone Joint Surg Am 2009;91(7):1683–8.

58. Reddy S, Pedowitz DI, Parekh SG, et al. The morbidity associated with osteochondral harvest from asymptomatic knees for the treatment of osteochondral lesions of the talus. Am J Sports Med 2007;35(1):80–5.

59. Woelfle JV, Reichel H, Javaheripour-Otto K, et al. Clinical outcome and magnetic resonance imaging after osteochondral autologous transplantation in osteochondritis dissecans of the talus. Foot Ankle Int 2013;34(2):173–9.

60. Gross CE, Adams SB, Easley ME, et al. Role of fresh osteochondral allografts for large talar osteochondral lesions. Instr Course Lect 2016;65:301–9.

61. Ahmad J, Jones K. Comparison of osteochondral autografts and allografts for treatment of recurrent or large talar osteochondral lesions. Foot Ankle Int 2016; 37(1):40–50.

62. Raikin SM. Fresh osteochondral allografts for large-volume cystic osteochondral defects of the talus. J Bone Joint Surg Am 2009;91(12):2818–26.

63. Haene R, Qamirani E, Story RA, et al. Intermediate outcomes of fresh talar osteochondral allografts for treatment of large osteochondral lesions of the talus. J Bone Joint Surg Am 2012;94(12):1105–10.

64. Hahn DB, Aanstoos ME, Wilkins RM. Osteochondral lesions of the talus treated with fresh talar allografts. Foot Ankle Int 2010;31(4):277–82.

65. Scott DJ, Steele J, Fletcher A, et al. Early outcomes of 3D printed total talus arthroplasty. Foot Ankle Spec 2019. [Epub ahead of print].

66. Giannini S, Vannini F. Operative treatment of osteochondral lesions of the talar dome: current concepts review. Foot Ankle Int 2004;25(3):168–75.

67. Phisitkul P, Akoh CC, Rungprai C, et al. Optimizing arthroscopy for osteochondral lesions of the talus: the effect of ankle positions and distraction during anterior and posterior arthroscopy in a cadaveric model. Arthroscopy 2017;33(12): 2238–45.

68. Van Dijk CN, Vuurberg G, Amendola A, et al. Anterior ankle arthroscopy: state of the art. J ISAKOS 2016;1(2):105–15.

69. Van Dijk CN, Vuurberg G, Batista J, et al. Posterior ankle arthroscopy: current state of the art. J ISAKOS 2017;2(5):269–77.

70. Orr JD, Dutton JH, Nelson JR, et al. Indications for and early complications associated with use of temporary invasive distraction for osteochondral graft transfer procedures for treatment of lateral osteochondral lesions of the talus. Foot Ankle Int 2014;35(1):50–5.

71. Kennedy JG, Murawski CD. The treatment of osteochondral lesions of the talus with autologous osteochondral transplantation and bone marrow aspirate concentrate. Cartilage 2011;2(4):327–36.

Posterior Ankle Impingement and Flexor Hallucis Longus Pathology

B. Dale Sharpe, DO[a], Brian D. Steginsky, DO[b,*],
Mallory Suhling, BS[c], Anand Vora, MD[c]

KEYWORDS

- Posterior ankle impingement • Os trigonum • Flexor hallucis longus
- Posterior ankle endoscopy • Dancing injuries

KEY POINTS

- Posterior ankle impingement syndrome results from recurrent trauma to the posterior ankle capsuloligamentous complex, flexor hallucis longus tendon, and/or os trigonum.
- Posterior ankle impingement syndrome often occurs in athletes that require dynamic or repetitive push-off maneuvers, including runners, tennis players, soccer players, and dancers.
- The complex and less familiar posterior ankle anatomy makes accurate identification and diagnosis difficult. MRI and differential injections are helpful to confirm the diagnosis.
- Nonsurgical treatment should include injections, physical therapy, and activity modification. Conservative treatment has been reported with success.
- When conservative treatment fails, the surgical approach must be thoughtfully contemplated to ensure that the underlying cause of posterior ankle pain is appropriately addressed.

INTRODUCTION

Posterior ankle pain is a common complaint, and the potential causative pathologic processes are diverse. The constellation of these numerous etiologies has been collectively referred to as posterior ankle impingement syndrome.[1] The pain associated with posterior ankle impingement is caused by bony or soft tissue impingement of the posterior ankle while in terminal plantar flexion. This condition is most frequently encountered in athletes who participate in sports that involve forceful, or repetitive, ankle plantar flexion.

The specific pathoanatomy can vary greatly for each patient, which has led to varying nomenclature. The intertwined, complex, deep posterior ankle structures limit

[a] Residency Program, OhioHealth Orthopedic Surgery, 5100 West Broad Street, Columbus, OH 43228, USA; [b] OhioHealth Orthopedic Surgeons, 303 East Town Street, Columbus, OH 43215, USA; [c] Illinois Bone and Joint Institute, LLC, 720 Florsheim Drive, Libertyville, IL 60048, USA
* Corresponding author.
E-mail address: Brian.steginsky@ohiohealth.com

Clin Sports Med 39 (2020) 911–930
https://doi.org/10.1016/j.csm.2020.06.001
0278-5919/20/© 2020 Elsevier Inc. All rights reserved.

sportsmed.theclinics.com

direct palpation and physical examination, making the diagnosis of posterior ankle impingement more difficult.[2] The treatment algorithms also have great variability dependent on the specific condition, sport, and season. This article discusses the associated pathology, diagnosis, conservative treatment, and surgical techniques associated with flexor hallucis longus (FHL) and posterior ankle impingement syndrome.

ANATOMY

The posterior ankle region consists of the bony and soft tissue structures positioned posterior to the tibiotalar joint, subtalar joint, and calcaneus. The posterior talar process constitutes the portion of the talus that extends posteriorly from the articular surface of the tibiotalar joint. This process consists of 2 projections, the posteromedial and posterolateral processes. The groove that lies between these posterior processes houses the FHL tendon (**Fig. 1**). The posterolateral process is referred to as the trigonal process and is more commonly implicated in posterior ankle impingement syndrome. When the trigonal process remains a nonfused entity from the talar body, it is referred to as the os trigonum.[2]

Os Trigonum

The os trigonum develops as a secondary ossification center and later undergoes fusion with the talar body via cartilaginous endochondral ossification in early adolescence. When mineralization and fusion are complete, an elongated posterolateral projection is called the Stieda process. The os trigonum represents a failure of the secondary ossification center to fully undergo fusion to the posterolateral talar process.[3] This failure of fusion of the ossific nucleus results in a fibrocartilage connection. The incidence has been reported to occur in 1.7% to 49% of the population, with most being asymptomatic.[4,5] The os trigonum is found to be present bilaterally in roughly 50% of cases.[6,7]

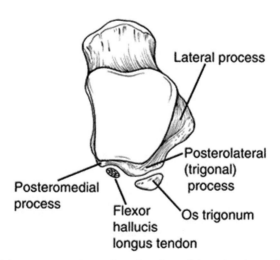

Fig. 1. Posterior talar process anatomy. Superior view of the talus shows the close relationship of the FHL tendon and trigonal process (os trigonum). (*From* Maquirriain J. Posterior Ankle Impingement Syndrome: *Journal of the American Academy of Orthopaedic Surgeons.* 2005;13(6):365-371; with permission.)

The specific contour and dimensions of the os trigonum are variable, but some generalizations can be made. It is most commonly triangular in shape, with an anterior, posterior, and inferior surface. The most common reports claim a size of 1 cm^2 as an estimate.[8] The anterior surface forms a fibrocartilaginous synchondrosis with the posterior lateral tubercle of the talus.[9] The posterior talofibular and posterior talocalcaneal ligaments arise from the posterior surface of the os trigonum.[9] The inferior surface often articulates with the posterior facet of the calcaneus. The FHL tendon courses just medial to the os trigonum, while its sheath is often attached to the medial os.[8]

Flexor Hallucis Longus

The origin of the FHL lies proximally on the posterior fibula and interosseous membrane. Distally, the tendon sheath forms a fibro-osseous tunnel that is attached to the posterior talus. The FHL tendon courses between the medial and lateral tubercles of the posterior talus.[9,10] The tendon continues beyond the posterior talus traveling plantar to the sustentaculum tali of the calcaneus. It then forms fibrous connections with the flexor digitorum longus tendon at the "Knot of Henry" as the FHL tendon crosses dorsally. The crossing of the FHL and flexor digitorum longus tendons occurs in the midfoot, plantar to the first tarsal-metatarsal joint. The FHL tendon continues to its insertion at the plantar base of the distal phalanx of the hallux.[11] The FHL functions primarily in active plantarflexion at the first metatarsophalangeal and hallux interphalangeal joints.[10]

PathoAnatomy: ETIOLOGY AND PATHOGENESIS

The potential causes of posterior ankle impingement syndrome are numerous. These include soft tissue injuries such as Achilles tendinopathy, retrocalcaneal bursitis, FHL tenosynovitis, FHL tendinitis; along with bony or osteochondral lesions such as bony impingement, Haglund's disease, stress fractures, osteochondritis dissecans, and tarsal coalitions. There are also neurovascular causes of posterior ankle pain including sural nerve entrapment, tarsal tunnel syndrome, and popliteal artery entrapment.[1]

Injury to the FHL tendon is one of the more common causes of posterior ankle pain. This injury is seen often in athletes that require dynamic, or repetitive, push-off maneuvers such runners, tennis players, and dancers. FHL tendinitis, or tenosynovitis, is the result of compression of the tendon within its sheath.[12] This entrapment can be the result of an aberrant, or low lying, FHL muscle belly, friction of the tendon with the os trigonum, and repetitive hyper plantarflexion leading to synovitis and synovial hypertrophy of the ankle and subtalar joints.[13] Tenosynovitis most commonly occurs within the fibro-osseous tunnel immediately posterior to the talus. This location places the tendon at the greatest risk, as the tendon travels within its sheath deep to the flexor retinaculum and between the posterior talar tubercles. This pathology is most commonly reported in dancers, but it also affects other athletes that rely on hyper plantarflexion such as soccer players, runners, ice skaters, and gymnasts.[14] Particularly in the case of ballet dancers, with en pointe positioning, plantar flexion may cause compression of the FHL tendon within the fibro-osseous tunnel. As the ankle progresses into a hyperplantar flexed position the talus internally rotates within the ankle mortise, relative to an externally rotated tibia.[15] This coupled rotation causes compression of the FHL tendon within the fibro-osseous tunnel that lies posteromedially. This compression leads to the development of tenosynovitis.[16] Furthermore, up to 12 times the body weight is transferred through the posterior ankle when a dancer is en pointe, explaining the high occurrence of posterior ankle pathology in dancers.[14,17]

Posterior impingement syndrome, or os trigonum syndrome, may be the result of acute fracture of Stieda process, os trigonum fracture, disruption of the fibrous connection from the posterior talus to the os, or injury to the posterior capsuloligamentous structures associated with the os trigonum.[18] The most common presentation of os trigonum syndrome is a patient with a sentinel episode of acute, forceful plantarflexion.[19] In the case of ballet dancers, this most commonly occurs in the en pointe and demi-pointe positions.[20] Hyper plantarflexion position allows the talus to rotate and become compressed between the superior calcaneus and the posterior distal tibia. This compression occurs secondary to the rotatory motion of the talus within the ankle mortise. With ankle dorsiflexion, the talus externally rotates, beneath a relatively internally rotated tibia, with the widest portion of the talar articular surface filling the ankle mortise, providing structural stability. While in plantarflexion, the talus internally rotates, beneath a relative externally rotated tibia, with a narrower region of the articular surface, allowing for some inherent instability.[15] This coupled rotation of the talus and distal tibia allows for the posterior talar process to compress between the calcaneus and tibia, causing bony impingement.

The pathologic processes that lead to pain are different in the case of acute injury versus chronic repetitive positioning. In the acute case, an elongated posterolateral talar tubercle (Stieda process) is compressed between the posterior malleolus and the calcaneus, causing fracture of the process or injury to the synchondrosis of the os trigonum.[21,22] In the chronic, or repetitive, plantarflexed positioning, both osseous and soft tissue structures are compressed in the posterior ankle. The posterior capsule and intra-articular synovium become irritated and initiate an inflammatory response. This response and the resultant edema leads to the development of pain and eventually permanent soft tissue change.[23] In addition to the capsule and synovium, the posterior talofibular and tibiotalar ligaments can develop fibrosis from repeated injury.[24,25] The transition to inflamed and fibrotic tissue ultimately limits range of motion, changing mechanics, and perpetuating the pathologic process (**Fig. 2**).

Multiple etiologies have been identified to result in soft tissue posterior ankle impingement. Liu and Mirzayan[26] reported a case of chronic posteromedial ankle impingement pain in the face of multiple inversion and eversion ankle sprains. Van Dijk and colleagues[27] also reported that significant traumatic lateral ankle sprains may result in medial ankle chondral compression injuries as well as partial rupture of the deep fibers of the posterior deep deltoid ligament. This pattern occurs as multiple lateral ligaments are torn, the ankle rotates out of the mortise allowing for the medial talar facet to come in contact with the medial malleolus. This can also cause tension failure of the posterior deep deltoid ligament. This pattern of injury can lead to hypertrophic synovitis and scar tissue formation that presents with subsequent posteromedial ankle impingement and pain.[27] In addition, the posterior tibiotalar ligament can become compressed between the medial malleolus and talar body.[1] The soft tissue impingement pattern most commonly presents with previous episodes of ankle instability and pain with the ankle in a plantar flexed position.

Posterolateral soft tissue impingement typically occurs secondary to fibrosis of an accessory ligament, the posterior intermalleolar ligament.[28] The posterior intermalleolar ligament spans the posterior ankle, from the malleolar fossa of the distal fibula to the posterior distal tibia cortex. The intermalleolar ligament is located between the posterior tibiofibular ligament (superior) and posterior talofibular ligament (inferior) and was found to be present in 56% of cadavers in one study.[28] With the ankle in a plantar flexed position, this accessory ligament can translate anteriorly into the posterior ankle joint, increasing the susceptibility to impingement and soft tissue injury.[1]

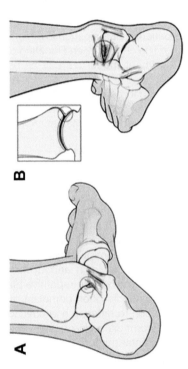

Fig. 2. (A) Illustration of posteromedial impingement, with entrapment of fibrotic scar tissue in the posteromedial ankle gutter (*circled*). (B) Illustration of posterolateral impingement, with the fibrotic soft tissue intra-articularly between the posterior tibiofibular and posterior talofibular ligaments. (*From* Giannini S, Buda R, Mosca M, Parma A, Di Caprio F. Posterior Ankle Impingement. *Foot Ankle Int.* 2013;34(3):459-465; with permission.)

Many athletes may attempt to compensate for their loss of plantar flexion, or painful plantar flexion, by using improper mechanics and positions. Dancers, specifically, will adopt an inverted en pointe or releve positions, referred to as sickling.[2] This adapted position minimizes posterior ankle impingement, however, it places the ankle in a relatively unstable position often lending to more anterolateral ankle sprains.[29] Other injuries often occur secondary to sickling, including calf strains, plantar foot pain, and toe curling.[2]

Concomitant pathologies are common in these populations. There is a high incidence of trigonal process injuries associated with FHL tenosynovitis in classic ballet dancers.[24] Treatment pathways can often be guided by presenting symptoms and sequentially eliminating the most common causes of posterior ankle pain.

CLINICAL PRESENTATION

The diagnosis and initial treatment is often based on clinical history. It is important for the clinician to inquire about the patient's participation in athletic activities and sport-specific foot and ankle positioning. The chronicity and location of pain, as well as success or failures with previous treatment modalities can all be helpful cues to the provider.

Hyper plantar flexion of the ankle and forceful push-off maneuvers, such as dancing, kicking, downhill running, or ambulation in heels may elicit pain.[1] The patient may describe mechanical symptoms associated with pain, such as "clicking," "popping," or "catching."

Patients may report increased pain with weight bearing and have discomfort with the push-off phase of the gait cycle. When the FHL is involved, the patient may report discomfort with motion of the first metatarsophalangeal joint.[30] Pain is often relieved with rest and controlled ankle motion, although this is not always the case.

The patient may report a history of ankle trauma, although symptoms may also be chronic.[2] In the case of an acute injury, such as a fracture of the posterolateral talar tubercle or injury to the synchondrosis, the clinician may elicit a history of a single traumatic hyper plantar flexion injury with resultant posterior ankle pain. Patients with os trigonum syndrome will often report similar pain and dysfunction, but frequently describe a more insidious onset of symptoms with repetitive plantar flexion.

In the case of FHL tenosynovitis, patients often complain of a longer duration of discomfort, and their pain can transition to differing anatomic locations. Patients will often complain of pain in the posteromedial ankle or the great toe, however, pain can be present at the plantar heel, plantar midfoot, or in concurrent locations.[10,14]

PHYSICAL EXAMINATION

Physical examination of the posterior ankle is frequently challenging, as the posterior ankle anatomy is complex, and posterior ankle pathology unrelated to the Achilles tendon is less frequently diagnosed. Therefore, a methodical approach to the physical examination is helpful. The patient should be examined in the prone position, in addition to standard supine or seated positions.

In the case of os trigonum syndrome, the unfused ossicle can often be palpated at the posterolateral aspect of the tibiotalar joint line. Soft tissue edema may also be visible and palpable in this region.[29] Passive range of motion of the ankle may be diminished, particularly in plantarflexion, with either chronic repetitive injury or acute fracture. This may be result of a mechanical block to motion and fibrosis, resulting from a chronic inflammatory process. The patient may also have reproducible pain at terminal plantar-flexion of the ankle; this has been referred to as the "nutcracker sign."[31]

Precise palpation along the course of the FHL tendon can provide important physical examination information, particularly because the tendon is palpable in multiple locations as it courses through the foot and ankle. The distal aspect of the tendon is palpable on the plantar aspect of the first metatarsophalangeal joint between the sesamoids. Moving proximally, it can be found at the Knot of Henry as it crosses the flexor digitorum longus tendon plantar to the medial cuneiform. In the medial hindfoot, the tendon can be palpated plantar to the sustentaculum of the calcaneus. The musculotendinous junction is often palpable at the posterior medial aspect of the ankle.[10] The point of maximal tenderness can direct the practitioner to the correct pathologic process. The physical examination finding of "pseudo hallux rigidus" is specific to FHL tenosynovitis, in which first metatarsophalangeal joint (MTPJ) dorsiflexion is limited when the ankle is in a neutral or dorsiflexed position.[13] However, MTPJ dorsiflexion improves when the ankle is positioned into plantarflexion. FHL tendon hypertrophy prevents the tendon from gliding into the fibro-osseous tunnel at the level of the talus when the ankle is neutral to dorsiflexed.[14]

IMAGING

Weight-bearing foot and ankle radiographs are mandatory before advance imaging is pursued. The os trigonum can be identified on the lateral radiograph (**Fig. 3**). The addition of radiographs in the lateral projection taken with 25° of external rotation may assist with the diagnosis of an os trigonum, as overlap with the posteromedial talar process is uncovered.[32] Acute fracture of an os trigonum, or Stieda process, can often be noted with an acute appearing fracture line or displacement of the posterior fragment. Weight-bearing ankle plantarflexion radiographs may demonstrate bony posterior ankle impingement.[33]

Computed tomography (CT) can be useful to aid in determining the spatial relationship of the os trigonum or prominent posterolateral process of the talus. CT imaging may also provide insight into any cystic formation or degenerative arthritis (**Fig. 4**). Bone scintigraphy (Technetium [Tc] 99) may be useful when CT cannot differentiate between a chronic fracture and an os trigonum. Increased uptake of the radiotracer is seen in patients with acute fractures of the trigonal process and with injury to the os trigonum synchondrosis. Patient's with an asymptomatic os trigonum do not

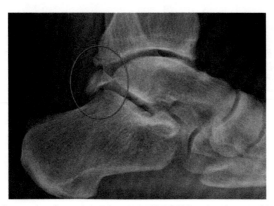

Fig. 3. Lateral radiograph of os trigonum, as indicated by circular marking. (*From* Carreira DS, Vora AM, Hearne KL, Kozy J. Outcome of Arthroscopic Treatment of Posterior Impingement of the Ankle. *Foot Ankle Int.* 2016;37(4):394-400; with permission.)

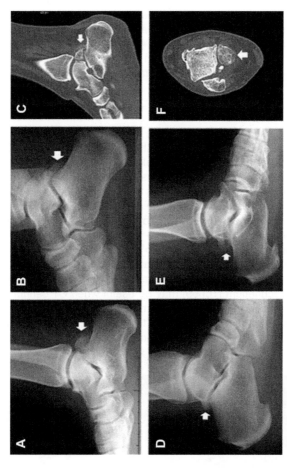

Fig. 4. Lateral views of the foot radiography demonstrate os trigonum (A) and Stieda process (B, D, E). The sagittal and coronal views of the computed tomographic scan demonstrate large os trigonum posterior to the talus (C, F). (*From* Carreira DS, Vora AM, Hearne KL, Kozy J. Outcome of Arthroscopic Treatment of Posterior Impingement of the Ankle. *Foot Ankle Int.* 2016;37(4):394-400; with permission.)

display any increased Tc 99 uptake. Diagnostically, a normal bone scan can effectively eliminate os trigonum syndrome.[9]

CT and bone scintigraphy cannot effectively evaluate the posterior ankle soft tissue anatomy as well as an MRI. Therefore, MRI has become the gold-standard diagnostic test for posterior ankle pathology.[34] MRI is helpful in diagnosing both acute and chronic pathologic processes, including trigonal arthritis, FHL tenosynovitis, ankle joint synovitis, and fracture (**Fig. 5**). Bone marrow edema may be evident in the posterior talar trigonal process, signifying the presence of microtrabecular fractures (without evidence of cortical disruption) from repetitive mechanical bony posterior impingement.[35] This bony edema may also be present within the synchondrosis of the os trigonum as visual evidence of a symptomatic os trigonum. MRI is also helpful to evaluate the FHL tendon (**Fig. 6**); however, care must be taken when interpreting FHL pathology on MRI, as there is a high incidence of intra-sheath effusions in asymptomatic patients.[36] In true cases of FHL tendinitis, intra-substance tendon enhancement will invariably be present. MRI has been shown to guide the patient's clinical course, as it aids in both diagnosis and treatment planning.[9]

CONSERVATIVE TREATMENT OPTIONS

With the exception of unstable acute fractures, initial nonsurgical treatment should be attempted for all patients. Patients with posterior ankle impingement often improve with rest alone.[2] In addition to rest and activity modification, standard conservative therapy typically consists of a combination of ice, elevation, nonsteroidal anti-inflammatory medications, and protected weight bearing and immobilization.[37] Immobilization is most commonly indicated in the case of acute injury or fracture.[38] Specific modes of immobilization have not been compared in the literature, but most authors suggest weight-bearing short leg cast or controlled ankle motion (CAM) walking boot. Physical therapy can also provide significant benefit with the appropriate pathology, or patients not improving with rest alone.[22] This course of therapy typically

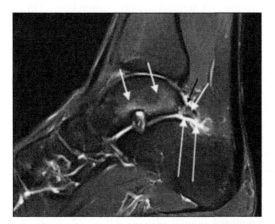

Fig. 5. (*A*) Sagittal T1-weighted MR image of Stieda process. (*B*) Sagittal T2-weighted MR image with fat suppression of Stieda process. (*C*) Sagittal T1-weighted MR image of large os trigonum. Note the loss of marrow continuity of the os with intact cortical margins. (*D*) Sagittal T2-weighted MR image with fat suppression. Note fluid surrounding the os. MR, magnetic resonance. (*From* Carreira DS, Vora AM, Hearne KL, Kozy J. Outcome of Arthroscopic Treatment of Posterior Impingement of the Ankle. *Foot Ankle Int.* 2016;37(4):394-400; with permission.)

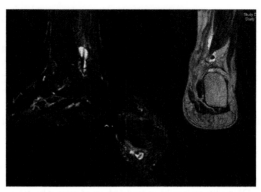

Fig. 6. Magnetic resonance imaging in the illustrated case showed tenosynovitis of the flexor hallucis longus at the posteromedial aspect of the ankle, whereas intraoperative findings showed synovitis and scarring at the posteromedial ankle instead of flexor hallucis longus tenosynovitis. (Lui TH. Arthroscopic Management of Posteromedial Ankle Impingement. Arthroscopy Techniques. Volume 4, Issue 5, October 2015, Pages e425-e427; with permission.)

consists of icing, ultrasound therapy, massage, and stretching to regain range of motion through diminishing the inflammatory process. Nonsurgical treatment has been reported to be successful in nearly 60% of patients.[38]

An adjunct to the conservative treatment pathway includes diagnostic injections with local anesthetics and/or corticosteroid. These injections are directed to the most symptomatic areas for each patient. The anesthetic can be placed within the soft tissues, tendon sheath, or intra-articular to aid in identifying the definitive cause of the patient's symptoms.[20] Posterior ankle impingement syndrome and FHL tendon pathology frequently coexist. Miyamoto and colleagues[39] suggested that multiple differential ultrasound guided injections to help localize the pathology. These investigators suggest an injection around the posterolateral talar process, followed by injection into the FHL tendon sheath 2-week later.[39] In addition to potential symptomatic relief, the use of injections may be used for diagnostic purposes prior to surgical intervention. The clinical improvement of symptoms has been reported in 84% of cases using combination of corticosteroid and local anesthetic.[22] Depending on the targeted location of the injection, fluoroscopic and ultrasound guidance have been used to achieve a more reproducible response.[40] There has been reported success with platelet-rich plasma injections in the treatment of tendinitis, however, there are not any published studies in relation to FHL tendinitis. This is the same scenario for mesenchymal stem cell injections. Many anecdotal reports have been made, but the authors are not aware of any comparative studies published regarding the subject manner of this article.

SURGICAL TREATMENT OPTIONS

Surgical treatment of posterior ankle impingement and/or FHL pathology is considered after conservative treatment course has proven to be unsuccessful, typically after 6 months of failed nonsurgical treatment. There are multiple strategies and techniques that have been reported to be successful in the surgical treatment of posterior ankle pain.

Open Procedures

Open approaches have long been the mainstay for surgical treatment of os trigonum syndrome and FHL pathology. Posterolateral and posteromedial approaches have been described and used with success. The posterolateral approach has traditionally been recommended for an isolated excision of an os trigonum, as it poses minimal risk to surrounding structures with appropriate exposure to remove the os. If the primary pathology is posterior bony impingement and/or involves the FHL tendon, a postero-medial approach is endorsed.[29,41]

Posterolateral

Patient is placed in the supine or lateral position with a thigh tourniquet on the operative leg. The incision is made in a linear fashion posterior to the distal fibula and medial to the peroneal tendons. Careful dissection is carried out in the superficial plane until the sural nerve has been identified and protected with retraction. Deep dissection continues to the posterior ankle capsule, and the capsule is incised in line with the dissection. The culprit os trigonum is then identified and removed with the use of rongeur or osteotome. This process can be facilitated with fluoroscopy. The rough bony surface is smoothed with the use of a rasp to prevent further soft tissue irritation. Bone wax should be applied to the exposed surface of posterior talus to aid in hemostasis. The entire wound is thoroughly irrigated with sterile saline and closure in a layered fashion.[41]

Posteromedial

The patient is placed in a supine position with a thigh tourniquet on the operative leg. The incision is made in a curvilinear fashion roughly 1-cm posterior to the medial malleolus. Superficial dissection concentrates to avoid injury to the superficial branches of the tibial nerve. Coetzee and colleagues[42] described the open approach through the interval between flexor digitorum longus and the neurovascular bundle. In this technique it is advised that if the surgeon is inexperienced with this approach, the interval between tibialis posterior and flexor digitorum longus can be used to place the neurovascular bundle further away from the dissection.[42] Deeper dissection reveals the superior flexor retinaculum, which is released in line with the skin incision. The FHL tendon sheath is routinely released to relieve any stenosis or tenosynovitis. The remaining flexor tendons and neurovascular bundle are then identified, mobilized, and gently retracted. The posterior ankle capsule is encountered and incised. The offending pathology is then treated as indicated.

The incision and dissection can be altered based on the pathology that is being treated with the operation. The incision should be placed more posteriorly if directing attention to the FHL tendon pathology, centering about 1-cm medial to Achilles tendon. Supine positioning with a bump placed beneath the contralateral hip will allow the operative lower extremity to externally rotate. Dissection is carried in an anterolateral direction toward the FHL tendon. The muscle belly of the FHL is identified and dissection is carried distally to ensure that the correct tendon has been identified. Once isolation of the tendon has been confirmed with hallux MTP and interphalangeal flexion, the FHL tendon sheath is identified and incised. The tibial nerve is not typically encountered during this altered approach as it remains out of the operative field when the FHL tendon is retracted medially to excise the os trigonum, removal of posterior bony impingement, or debridement of the FHL tendon or fibro-osseous tunnel at the posterior talus.[41] This approach also minimizes the risk of subsequent peroneal tendinitis and adhesion that has been reported with the posterolateral approach.[38]

Endoscopic Approaches

Ankle arthroscopic techniques have been at a steady growth as it has been shown to provide advantages in minimizing postoperative scarring and fibrosis that results from open procedures. These procedures also decrease postoperative pain secondary to minimal soft tissue disruption.[43] In the setting of posterior impingement syndrome, the arthroscopic instruments and techniques are used within extra-capsular soft tissues, denoting this as an endoscopic procedure[44] (**Figs. 7** and **8**). Van Dijk and colleagues[45] described and published the surgical techniques of hindfoot endoscopy

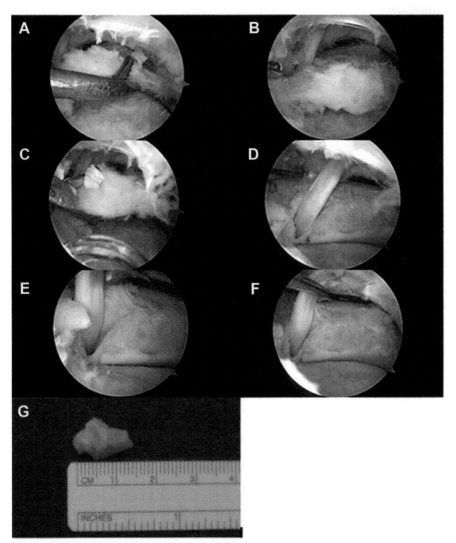

Fig. 7. Endoscopic excision of os trigonum. Debridement of the retrocalcaneal bursa reveals the posterior capsule and ligamentous complex. The posterior talofibular ligament is released to aid in mobilizing the os trigonum (*A*). The borders of the os trigonum are outlined with debridement of the surrounding soft tissue (*B*). The os is excised with arthroscopic graspers after the synchondrosis has been disrupted with an elevator or osteotome (*C*). The FHL tendon is then evaluated for tenosynovitis and/or tearing (*D*). The fibro-osseous tunnel is also inspected for signs of stenosis (*E*). The posterior aspects of the tibiotalar and subtalar joints can be inspected for osteochondral lesions or loose bodies (*F*). The triangular shaped os of typical size (1.5 cm) is displayed on the back table (*G*).

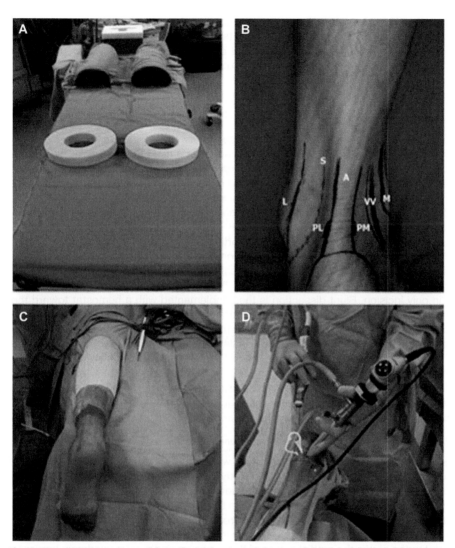

Fig. 8. Standard posterior ankle arthroscopy is demonstrated (*A*), and patient is placed in the prone position with thigh tourniquet and the foot is at the end of the bed (*C*). Surface anatomy shows posterolateral (PL), posteromedial (PM), Achilles tendon (A), medial malleolus (M), lateral malleolus (L), sural nerve (S), and tibial nerve and vessels (VV) (*B*). A 4.0-mm, 30° arthroscope is inserted in the PL portal, the shaver is inserted in the PM portal, and the surgeon can dorsiflex the ankle joint by leaning the surgeon's body forward (*D*). (*From* Rungprai C, Tennant JN, Phisitkul P. Disorders of the Flexor Hallucis Longus and Os Trigonum. *Clinics in Sports Medicine.* 2015;34(4):741-759; with permission.)

in numerous accounts to lay the groundwork for the progression and success of these procedures.

The most common positioning for this procedure places the patient prone on the operative table. A thigh tourniquet is again placed on the operative extremity. The patient is also placed on the table so that the ankle is allowed to dorsiflex either with placement of bumps or bolsters or allowing the foot to hang from the end of the operative table. Distraction is not routinely used for these procedures. The prone posterior approach is a more direct approach than a described lateral approach that can be performed with the patient in a lateral decubitus position.[46,47] This more direct approach minimizes the risk to the anatomic structures medial and lateral to the posterior ankle. The FHL pathology can also be addressed more simply from the prone position, similar in manner to the posteromedial open approach.

Establishing Portals

Before establishing portal placement, the superficial anatomic structures are marked on the skin. These typically include medial and lateral malleoli, superior portion of the calcaneal tuberosity, medial and lateral borders of Achilles tendon, the posteromedial neurovascular bundle, and the sural nerve laterally. Given that the approach is extra-articular, calf or thigh tourniquet is recommended, as small vessels will continue to bleed as fluid pressure does provide the same level of tamponade when compared to an intra-articular procedure.

The posteromedial and posterolateral portals mirror each other just off the border of either side of the Achilles tendon. These portals are placed about 1.5 cm proximal to the superior margin of the calcaneal tuberosity, just superior to a horizontal line at the level of the distal extent of the distal fibula.[45] The lateral portal is established first with skin only incision. Blunt dissection is then implemented with a hemostat toward the webspace between the first and second toes to provide a soft tissue defect to be replaced by the trocar and arthroscope. The 30°arthroscope is then placed in the posterolateral portal to the posterior ankle capsule, remaining extra-articular. The posteromedial portal is then established in the same fashion previously described with the hemostat clamp directed toward the arthroscope shaft. The hemostat is then guided along the arthroscope to the posterior ankle. All instruments that are passed through the posteromedial portal are exchanged in this same fashion, following the shaft of the arthroscope.[45]

Details of the Endoscopic Surgical Procedure

Nearly all hindfoot endoscopic procedures will begin with an initial debridement of the posterior ankle retrocalcaneal bursa and fatty tissue to allow for improved visualization for the indicated procedure. Careful attention must be paid in this step to hemostasis to maintain the acquired visualization. Deep to the debrided bursa and fatty tissue, the os trigonum will be identified as the most prominent posterior bony structure. The FHL tendon can be identified most reliably proximal and medial to the os trigonum.[41] The FHL tendon marks the medial extent of the exposure and can be used as a barrier to protect the posteromedial neurovascular structures. The tendon identity can be confirmed with motion at the first interphalangeal and MTPJ, which should elicit gliding of the tendon that can be visualized through the arthroscope. Following this identification and initial debridement, the os trigonum can then be mobilized with debridement of all tissue surrounding the os, including detachment of the posterior talofibular ligament, the talocalcaneal ligament, and the flexor retinaculum.[45]

If planning to excise the os trigonum, the fibrous synchondrosis must be identified. This can be accomplished with the use of an arthroscopic probe. A small periosteal elevator, or freer, can then be placed within this established space to lever the os trigonum from its attachment to the posterior talus. Once the os trigonum has been mobilized adequately, a grasper can be inserted and the os can be removed. If the os trigonum is too large in size, or difficult to mobilize, it can also be excised in a piecemeal fashion. The remaining posterior talus should be inspected following removal of the os trigonum, as posterior bony impingement may still be present and should be addressed. To this same point, the remaining posterior talus may be prominent enough to irritate the FHL tendon and additional debridement, or exostectomy, should ensue. Aggressive use of a rotary bur may predispose to the formation of ossification in the posterior ankle tissues, as fluid lavage cannot remove all debris related to use of the burr.

FHL tendon pathology can also be addressed with this same endoscopic approach. Once the os trigonum has been excised, the FHL tendon can be examined with more detail. Allowing the ankle to range from full plantarflexion to dorsiflexion, along with motion of the first MTP joint, will demonstrate full visualization of the FHL excursion. Damage to the FHL tendon, including partial tearing and surrounding tenosynovitis, can be debrided with the arthroscopic shaver. If there is impingement of the FHL tendon or stenosis within the fibro-osseous tunnel during range of motion, this can also be debrided to allow for uninhibited gliding. If the compression of the tendon is too great within this tunnel, the tunnel and FHL retinaculum can be released from the posterior talar process with arthroscopic scissors.[45] If a tear is identified and determined to be greater than 50% of the tendon, the surgeon should proceed with repair of the tendon, with either open or arthroscopic techniques.[41] The conclusion of the procedure should result in visualized full excursion of the FHL tendon without compression or remaining damage to the tendon.

The posterior aspect of the ankle and subtalar articular surfaces can also be examined following the previously described portions of the procedure. Any intra-articular synovitis or loose bodies can be identified and debrided when visualized. Cartilage defects can also be debrided and or microfractured via this posterior approach as well. The ankle can be manipulated to allow for better visualization, anterior drawer maneuver aids in creating space for instrument maneuvering within the joint.[41]

POSTOPERATIVE PROTOCOL

Protocols vary depending on the pathology present, concomitant procedures, and open versus endoscopic approaches. Generally, patients are typically placed in a well-padded splint, or soft dressing with CAM walker boot, with the ankle in neutral position in the operating room. The patient remains non–weight bearing for roughly 7 to 14 days, or until the skin incisions have matured sufficiently. Patient are then transitioned to a CAM walker boot with the goal of gait progression and weight bearing as tolerated.[48]

Patients participate in early range of motion exercises including passive, active-assist, and active techniques. This is frequently performed independently, and formal physical therapy is prescribed when deemed necessary. Reestablishing full dorsiflexion is the primary focus of this early motion protocol, in attempt to prevent fibrosis or adhesions from the local surgical trauma to posterior soft tissues. This early motion protocol is initiated earlier with endoscopic techniques, as the soft tissue disruption and time to heal incisions is less than open techniques. Patients begin to progress to regular shoe wear when they have achieved a painless standard gait in the CAM walker boot. This most commonly occurs between 2 and 3 weeks postoperatively. At the time of regular shoe wear, physical therapy for ankle strengthening and sport-specific training is initiated. This rehabilitation phase progresses as symptoms and response to therapy allow. Patients are generally released to return to full activity and sports competition around 6 weeks postoperatively.[48]

CLINICAL OUTCOMES

The clinical outcomes and reported success of conservative therapy is incredibly variable throughout the literature. The effectiveness depends as much on the patient, their physical demands, as the prescribed nonoperative treatment regimen. Symptoms have been shown to be improved in patients involved in lower demand activities, while patients participated in higher demand activities have higher rates of symptom recurrence.[29,49] Particularly related to os trigonum syndrome, success rates for conservative therapy have been reported as 60% to 84%.[22,38]

The reported success rates of corticosteroid and/or local anesthetic injections have also been shown to vary greatly. These rates have ranged from 29% to 100%.[22,38] Injections have been shown to aid in confirming the definitive diagnosis causing the patients' symptoms.[40] These reports have also made the recommendation that these injections should not be performed without guidance, in the form of fluoroscopy or ultrasound, or in quick succession secondary to the risk of tendon rupture or soft tissue damage.[33]

Open approaches for the excision of os trigonum have been found to be successful for the patients in which the os is truly the culprit of the symptoms.[29,50] Open excision of os trigonum was found to produce good to excellent results in 88% of patients in one series.[38] In a later reported series of dancers, 26 open procedures were performed for FHL tendinitis and posterior impingement, 9 for isolated tendinitis, and 6 for isolated posterior impingement syndrome. The authors reported good to excellent results in 76% of cases, with unrestricted return to dance 5 months following the operation for posterior impingement.[24] The decision for posteromedial versus posterolateral approach should be driven by the patient pathology and the preference of the surgeon. The literature has demonstrated improvement in American Orthopaedic Food and Ankle Society (AOFAS) scores and a return to full activity between 3 and 6 months after surgery.[43,51]

Endoscopic treatment has also been shown to provide relief and early return to activity reliably in patients with os trigonum syndrome and posterior impingement. In a reported series of 16 posterior ankle endoscopic procedures evaluated at a mean follow-up of 32 months, all patients reported good to excellent health-related quality of life and functional outcome scores, with 93% return to preinjury athletic level.[52] In the largest series of endoscopic treatment of posterior ankle impingement, Scholten demonstrated improvement in AOFAS scores in 55 patients from 75 to 90.[53] This group also noted that 84% and 68% of these patients rated their results to be good or excellent, respectively. In the largest series of patients with os trigonum syndrome, Carreira and colleagues[48] reported improved Visual Analog Scale pain scores, AOFAS Hindfoot scores, and unchanged Tegner Activity scores in 20 athletes treated with endoscopic treatment of posterior impingement syndrome. All motion variables were found to be statistically similar between the affected and unaffected sides. In comparing preoperative and postoperative range of motion of the affected side, only plantarflexion was found to be significant gain in motion.[48] Outcomes have also shown significantly improved AOFAS scores.[54,55] Return to activity and sports have been reported between 6 weeks and 6 months.[43,52,55]

Conservative treatment has been found to be successful in the treatment of FHL stenosing tenosynovitis in 46% to 64% of patients at 1 year.[10] There has been a high reported rate of recurrence, however.[56] It has also be reported that as many as 13% of these patients were ultimately found to have a longitudinal tear of the FHL tendon.[57] When conservative treatment does not provide the desire relief, or patients have episodes of recurrence that prevent functional activity, surgical intervention may be recommended. Surgical treatment, including debridement of FHL tendon along with the release of the retinaculum and the fibro-osseous tunnel, has been shown to be effective through both open and endoscopic approaches. Patient satisfaction has been reported between 85% and 90% with open surgery and 80% with arthroscopic surgery.[13,14,57] Patients have reported full return to sports activity in 81% to 100% of cases, after either open or arthroscopic procedures.[13,16,24,54] Return to sport activity has been shorter, 6 to 8 weeks, with endoscopic approach when compared with open surgery, 12 to 25 weeks.[16,24,54,58]

COMPLICATIONS

Iatrogenic injury resulting in later complications has been reported for these surgical procedures, albeit at relatively low rates. Sural nerve injury is of concern with both open and endoscopic posterolateral approaches. This injury is most commonly result of improper portal placement, poor placement of arthroscopic instruments, and excessive dissection and retraction in open procedures. Sural nerve injury has been reported to be 3.4% to 8.3% with endoscopic procedures and 6.3% to 19.5% with open surgery.[43,46,51,54,59–61]

Procedures for medial pathology, both endoscopic and posteromedial open approach, have the potential to result in injury to the medial neurovascular bundle. The incidence of tibial nerve injury has been reported in 6.7% of open and 11.1% of endoscopic procedures.[13,29] These particular patient cohorts showed full recovery of nerve function within 1 year of surgery.[29]

Infectious complications related to arthroscopic surgery has reported incidence, ranging from 3.3% to 6.7% for superficial and 3.3% for deep infections.[29,46] Open procedure infection rates have been shown at 2.4% of cases.

SUMMARY

Posterior ankle pain can be attributed to numerous causes, including posterior ankle bony and soft tissue impingement, FHL pathology, and symptomatic os trigonum. Posterior ankle pain most commonly occurs in patients that perform repetitive ankle plantarflexion exercises, such as dancers, tennis players, and soccer players. Differentiating the precise cause of posterior ankle pain can be challenging for the physician. A well-performed history and physical examination often cues the clinician into the etiology of posterior ankle pain. However, advanced imaging (MRI and CT) and differential diagnostic injections (with or without ultrasound) can assist with a more accurate diagnosis. Conservative treatment should include a combination of rest, immobilization, injections, and physical therapy. Surgery may be considered after 6-month of failed conservative treatment. Generally, outcomes are excellent.

DISCLOSURE

The authors have nothing to disclose.

REFERENCES

1. Giannini S, Buda R, Mosca M, et al. Posterior ankle impingement. Foot Ankle Int 2013;34(3):459–65.
2. Maquirriain J. Posterior ankle impingement syndrome. J Am Acad Orthop Surg 2005;13(6):365–71.
3. Grogan DP, Walling AK, Ogden JA. Anatomy of the os trigonum. J Pediatr Orthop 1990;10(5):618–22.
4. Mann R, Owsley D. Os trigonum. Variation of a common accessory ossicle of the talus. J Am Podiatr Med Assoc 1990;80(10):536–9.

5. Kose O, Okan A, Durakbasa M, et al. Fracture of the os trigonum: a case report. J Orthop Surg (Hong Kong) 2006;14(3):354–6.

6. Lawson JP. Symptomatic radiographic variants in extremities. Radiology 1985; 157(3):625–31.

7. Heyer JH, Rose DJ. Os trigonum excision in dancers via an open posteromedial approach. Foot Ankle Int 2017;38(1):27–35.

8. Davies M. The os trigonum syndrome. Foot 2004;14(3):119–23.

9. Karasick D, Schweitzer ME. The os trigonum syndrome: imaging features. Am J Roentgenol 1996;166(1):125–9.

10. Michelson J, Dunn L. Tenosynovitis of the flexor hallucis longus: a clinical study of the spectrum of presentation and treatment. Foot Ankle Int 2005;26(4):291–303.

11. O'Sullivan E, Carare-Nnadi R, Greenslade J, et al. Clinical significance of variations in the interconnections between flexor digitorum longus and flexor hallucis longus in the region of the knot of Henry. Clin Anat 2005;18(2):121–5.

12. Jones DC. Tendon disorders of the foot and ankle. J Am Acad Orthop Surg 1993; 1(2):87–94.

13. Corte-Real NM, Moreira RM, Guerra-Pinto F. Arthroscopic treatment of tenosynovitis of the flexor hallucis longus tendon. Foot Ankle Int 2012;33(12):1108–12.

14. Hamilton WG. Stenosing tenosynovitis of the flexor hallucis longus tendon and posterior impingement upon the os trigonum in ballet dancers. Foot Ankle 1982;3(2):74–80.

15. Brockett CL, Chapman GJ. Biomechanics of the ankle. Orthop Trauma 2016; 30(3):232–8.

16. Kolettis GJ, Micheli LJ, Klein JD. Release of the flexor hallucis longus tendon in ballet dancers*. J Bone Joint Surg 1996;78(9):1386–90.

17. Macintyre J, Joy E. Foot and ankle injuries in dance. Clin Sports Med 2000;19(2): 351–68.

18. Nault M-L, Kocher MS, Micheli LJ. Os trigonum syndrome. J Am Acad Orthop Surg 2014;22(9):545–53.

19. Ihle CL, Cochran RM. Fracture of the fused os trigonum. Am J Sports Med 1982; 10(1):47–50.

20. Brodsky AE, Khalil MA. Talar compression syndrome. Am J Sports Med 1986; 14(6):472–6.

21. Shepherd FJ. A hitherto undescribed fracture of the astragalus. J Anat Physiol 1882;17(Pt 1):79–81.

22. Mouhsine E, Djahangiri A, Garofalo R. Fracture of the non fused os trigonum, a rare cause of hindfoot pain. A case report and review of the literature. Chir Organi Mov 2004;89(2):171–5.

23. Howse AJG. Posterior block of the ankle joint in dancers. Foot Ankle 1982; 3(2):81–4.

24. Hamilton WG, Geppert MJ, Thompson FM. Pain in the posterior aspect of the ankle in dancers. differential diagnosis and operative treatment*. J Bone Joint Surg 1996;78(10):1491–500.

25. Russell JA, Kruse DW, Koutedakis Y, et al. Pathoanatomy of posterior ankle impingement in ballet dancers. Clin Anat 2010;23(6):613–21.

26. Liu SH, Mirzayan R. Posteromedial ankle impingement. Arthroscopy 1993;9(6): 709–11.

27. van Dijk CN, Bossuyt PM, Marti RK. Medial ankle pain after lateral ligament rupture. J Bone Joint Surg Br 1996;78(4):562–7.

28. Rosenberg ZS, Cheung YY, Beltran J, et al. Posterior intermalleolar ligament of the ankle: normal anatomy and MR imaging features. Am J Roentgenol 1995; 165(2):387–90.

29. Marotta JJ, Micheli LJ. Os trigonum impingement in dancers. Am J Sports Med 1992;20(5):533–6.

30. Gould N. Stenosing tenosynovitis of the flexor hallucis longus tendon at the great toe. Foot Ankle 1981;2(1):46–8.

31. Georgiannos D, Bisbinas I. Endoscopic versus open excision of os trigonum for the treatment of posterior ankle impingement syndrome in an athletic population: a randomized controlled study with 5-year follow-up. Am J Sports Med 2017; 45(6):1388–94.

32. Wiegerinck JI, Vroemen JC, van Dongen TH, et al. The posterior impingement view: an alternative conventional projection to detect bony posterior ankle impingement. Arthroscopy 2014;30(10):1311–6.

33. Blake R, Lallas P, Ferguson H. The os trigonum syndrome. A literature review. J Am Podiatr Med Assoc 1992;82(3):154–61.

34. Wakeley CJ, Johnson DP, Watt I. The value of MR imaging in the diagnosis of the os trigonum syndrome. Skeletal Radiol 1996;25(2):133–6.

35. Bureau NJ, Cardinal É, Hobden R, et al. Posterior ankle impingement syndrome: MR imaging findings in seven patients. Radiology 2000;215(2):497–503.

36. Link SC, Erickson SJ, Timins ME. MR imaging of the ankle and foot: normal structures and anatomic variants that may simulate disease. Am J Roentgenol 1993; 161(3):607–12.

37. Rogers J, Dijkstra P, Mccourt P, et al. Posterior ankle impingement syndrome: a clinical review with reference to horizontal jump athletes. Acta Orthop Belg 2010;76(5):572–9.

38. Hedrick MR, McBryde AM. Posterior ankle impingement. Foot Ankle Int 1994; 15(1):2–8.

39. Miyamoto W, Takao M, Matsushita T. Hindfoot endoscopy for posterior ankle impingement syndrome and flexor hallucis longus tendon disorders. Foot Ankle Clin 2015;20(1):139–47.

40. Jones DM, Saltzman CL, El-Khoury G. The diagnosis of the os trigonum syndrome with a fluoroscopically controlled injection of local anesthetic. Iowa Orthop J 1999;19:122–6.

41. Rungprai C, Tennant JN, Phisitkul P. Disorders of the flexor hallucis longus and os trigonum. Clin Sports Med 2015;34(4):741–59.

42. Coetzee JC, Seybold JD, Moser BR, et al. Management of posterior impingement in the ankle in athletes and dancers. Foot Ankle Int 2015;36(8):988–94.

43. Guo QW, Hu YL, Jiao C, et al. Open versus endoscopic excision of a symptomatic os trigonum: a comparative study of 41 cases. Arthroscopy 2010;26(3): 384–90.

44. van Dijk CN. Hindfoot endoscopy for posterior ankle pain. Instr Course Lect 2006; 55:545–54.

45. van Dijk C, de Leeuw P, Scholten P. Hindfoot endoscopy for posterior ankle impingement. J Bone Joint Surg Am 2009;91:287–98.

46. Galla M, Lobenhoffer P. Technique and results of arthroscopic treatment of posterior ankle impingement. Foot Ankle Surg 2011;17(2):79–84.

47. Park CH, Kim SY, Kim JR, et al. Arthroscopic excision of a symptomatic os trigonum in a lateral decubitus position. Foot Ankle Int 2013;34(7):990–4.

48. Carreira DS, Vora AM, Hearne KL, et al. Outcome of arthroscopic treatment of posterior impingement of the ankle. Foot Ankle Int 2016;37(4):394–400.

49. Rathur S, Clifford PD, Chapman CB. Posterior ankle impingement: os trigonum syndrome. Am J Orthop 2009;38(5):252–3.

50. Wredmark T, Carlstedt CA, Bauer H, et al. Os trigonum syndrome: a clinical entity in ballet dancers. Foot Ankle 1991;11(6):404–6.

51. Abramowitz Y, Wollstein R, Barzilay Y, et al. Outcome of resection of a symptomatic os trigonum. J Bone Joint Surg Am 2003;85(6):1051–7.

52. Willits K, Sonneveld H, Amendola A, et al. Outcome of posterior ankle arthroscopy for hindfoot impingement. Arthroscopy 2008;24(2):196–202.

53. Scholten P, Sierevelt I, van Dijk C. Hindfoot endoscopy for posterior ankle impingement. J Bone Joint Surg Am 2008;90(12):2665–72.

54. Ahn JH, Kim Y-C, Kim H-Y. Arthroscopic versus posterior endoscopic excision of a symptomatic Os trigonum: a retrospective cohort study. Am J Sports Med 2013; 41(5):1082–9.

55. Calder JD, Sexton SA, Pearce CJ. Return to training and playing after posterior ankle arthroscopy for posterior impingement in elite professional soccer. Am J Sports Med 2010;38(1):120–4.

56. Solomon R, Solomon J, Minton SC. Preventing dance injuries. 2nd edition. Champaign (IL): Human Kinetics; 2005.

57. Sammarco GJ, Cooper PS. Flexor hallucis longus tendon injury in dancers and nondancers. Foot Ankle Int 1998;19(6):356–62.

58. Theodoropoulos JS, Wolin PM, Taylor DW. Arthroscopic release of flexor hallucis longus tendon using modified posteromedial and posterolateral portals in the supine position. Foot 2009;19(4):218–21.

59. Noguchi H, Ishii Y, Takeda M, et al. Arthroscopic excision of posterior ankle bony impingement for early return to the field: short-term results. Foot Ankle Int 2010; 31(5):398–403.

60. Ogut T, Ayhan E, Irgit K, et al. Endoscopic treatment of posterior ankle pain. Knee Surg Sports Traumatol Arthrosc 2011;19(8):1355–61.

61. Tey M, Monllau JC, Centenera JM, et al. Benefits of arthroscopic tuberculoplasty in posterior ankle impingement syndrome. Knee Surg Sports Traumatol Arthrosc 2007;15(10):1235–9.

Statement of Ownership, Management, and Circulation
UNITED STATES POSTAL SERVICE® (All Periodicals Publications Except Requester Publications)

1. Publication Title	2. Publication Number	3. Filing Date
CLINICS IN SPORTS MEDICINE	000 – 702	9/18/2020

4. Issue Frequency	5. Number of Issues Published Annually	6. Annual Subscription Price
JAN, APR, JUL, OCT	4	$364.00

7. Complete Mailing Address of Known Office of Publication *(Not printer) (Street, city, county, state, and ZIP+4®)*

ELSEVIER INC.
230 Park Avenue, Suite 800
New York, NY 10169

Contact Person
Malathi Samayan

Telephone *(Include area code)*
91-44-4299-4507

8. Complete Mailing Address of Headquarters or General Business Office of Publisher *(Not printer)*

ELSEVIER INC.
230 Park Avenue, Suite 800
New York, NY 10169

9. Full Names and Complete Mailing Addresses of Publisher, Editor, and Managing Editor *(Do not leave blank)*

Publisher *(Name and complete mailing address)*

TAYLOR BALL, ELSEVIER INC.
1600 JOHN F KENNEDY BLVD. SUITE 1800
PHILADELPHIA, PA 19103-2899

Editor *(Name and complete mailing address)*

LAUREN BOYLE, ELSEVIER INC.
1600 JOHN F KENNEDY BLVD. SUITE 1800
PHILADELPHIA, PA 19103-2899

Managing Editor *(Name and complete mailing address)*

PATRICK MANLEY, ELSEVIER INC.
1600 JOHN F KENNEDY BLVD. SUITE 1800
PHILADELPHIA, PA 19103-2899

10. Owner *(Do not leave blank. If the publication is owned by a corporation, give the name and address of the corporation immediately followed by the names and addresses of all stockholders owning or holding 1 percent or more of the total amount of stock. If not owned by a corporation, give the names and addresses of the individual owners. If owned by a partnership or other unincorporated firm, give its name and address as well as those of each individual owner. If the publication is published by a nonprofit organization, give its name and address.)*

Full Name	Complete Mailing Address
WHOLLY OWNED SUBSIDIARY OF REED/ELSEVIER, US HOLDINGS	1600 JOHN F KENNEDY BLVD. SUITE 1800 PHILADELPHIA, PA 19103-2899

11. Known Bondholders, Mortgagees, and Other Security Holders Owning or Holding 1 Percent or More of Total Amount of Bonds, Mortgages, or Other Securities. If none, check box ▶ ☐ None

Full Name	Complete Mailing Address
N/A	

12. Tax Status *(For completion by nonprofit organizations authorized to mail at nonprofit rates) (Check one)*
The purpose, function, and nonprofit status of this organization and the exempt status for federal income tax purposes:
☒ Has Not Changed During Preceding 12 Months
☐ Has Changed During Preceding 12 Months *(Publisher must submit explanation of change with this statement)*

PS Form **3526**, July 2014 *(Page 1 of 4 (see instructions page 4))* PSN: 7530-01-000-9931 PRIVACY NOTICE: See our privacy policy on www.usps.com.

13. Publication Title			14. Issue Date for Circulation Data Below
CLINICS IN SPORTS MEDICINE			JULY 2020

15. Extent and Nature of Circulation			Average No. Copies Each Issue During Preceding 12 Months	No. Copies of Single Issue Published Nearest to Filing Date
a. Total Number of Copies *(Net press run)*			179	171
b. Paid Circulation (By Mail and Outside the Mail)	(1)	Mailed Outside-County Paid Subscriptions Stated on PS Form 3541 (Include paid distribution above nominal rate, advertiser's proof copies, and exchange copies)	111	99
	(2)	Mailed In-County Paid Subscriptions Stated on PS Form 3541 (Include paid distribution above nominal rate, advertiser's proof copies, and exchange copies)	0	0
	(3)	Paid Distribution Outside the Mails Including Sales Through Dealers and Carriers, Street Vendors, Counter Sales, and Other Paid Distribution Outside USPS®	34	38
	(4)	Paid Distribution by Other Classes of Mail Through the USPS (e.g., First-Class Mail®)	0	0
c. Total Paid Distribution *(Sum of 15b (1), (2), (3), and (4))*		▶	145	137
d. Free or Nominal Rate Distribution (By Mail and Outside the Mail)	(1)	Free or Nominal Rate Outside-County Copies included on PS Form 3541	20	18
	(2)	Free or Nominal Rate In-County Copies included on PS Form 3541	0	0
	(3)	Free or Nominal Rate Copies Mailed at Other Classes Through the USPS (e.g., First-Class Mail)	0	0
	(4)	Free or Nominal Rate Distribution Outside the Mail (Carriers or other means)	20	18
e. Total Free or Nominal Rate Distribution *(Sum of 15d (1), (2), (3) and (4))*		▶	20	18
f. Total Distribution *(Sum of 15c and 15e)*		▶	165	155
g. Copies not Distributed *(See Instructions to Publishers #4 (page #3))*		▶	14	16
h. Total *(Sum of 15f and g)*		▶	179	171
i. Percent Paid *(15c divided by 15f times 100)*		▶	87.87%	88.39%

* If you are claiming electronic copies, go to line 16 on page 3. If you are not claiming electronic copies, skip to line 17 on page 3.

16. Electronic Copy Circulation	Average No. Copies Each Issue During Preceding 12 Months	No. Copies of Single Issue Published Nearest to Filing Date
a. Paid Electronic Copies ▶		
b. Total Paid Print Copies (Line 15c) + Paid Electronic Copies (Line 16a) ▶		
c. Total Print Distribution (Line 15f) + Paid Electronic Copies (Line 16a) ▶		
d. Percent Paid (Both Print & Electronic Copies) (16b divided by 16c × 100) ▶		

☒ I certify that 50% of all my distributed copies (electronic and print) are paid above a nominal price.

17. Publication of Statement of Ownership

☒ If the publication is a general publication, publication of this statement is required. Will be printed in the OCTOBER 2020 issue of this publication. ☐ Publication not required.

18. Signature and Title of Editor, Publisher, Business Manager, or Owner

Malathi Samayan

Malathi Samayan - Distribution Controller

Date 9/18/2020

I certify that all information furnished on this form is true and complete. I understand that anyone who furnishes false or misleading information on this form or who omits material or information requested on the form may be subject to criminal sanctions (including fines and imprisonment) and/or civil sanctions (including civil penalties).

PS Form **3526**, July 2014 *(Page 3 of 4)* PRIVACY NOTICE: See our privacy policy on www.usps.com

Printed and bound by CPI Group (UK) Ltd, Croydon, CR0 4YY

08/05/2025

01864691-0001